THE

*J*offrey
*B*allet *S*chool's

BALLET-FIT

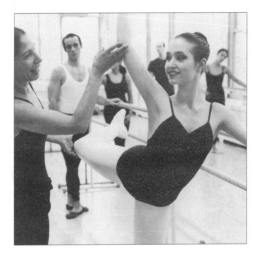

ST. MARTIN'S GRIFFIN
NEW YORK

THE
Joffrey
Ballet School's
BALLET-FIT

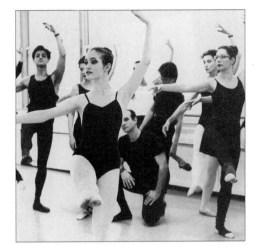

DENA SIMONE MOSS
ALLISON KYLE LEOPOLD

WITH PHOTOGRAPHS BY
STEVE LADNER

BOOK DESIGN BY LYNNE AMFT

Photographs © 1998 by Steve Ladner, used by permission
Makeup by M.A.C.

Library of Congress Cataloging-in-Publication Data
Leopold, Allison Kyle.
The Joffrey Ballet School's ballet-fit / Allison Kyle Leopold,
Dena Simone Moss ; [photographs by Steve Ladner]. —1st ed.
p.   cm.
Includes bibliographical references (p.   ) and index.
ISBN 0-312-19470-6
1. Ballet dancing. 2. Ballet—Study and teaching. 3. Physical fitness.
4. Joffrey Ballet School. I. Moss, Dena Simone. II. Joffrey Ballet School. III. Title.
GV1788.M67   1998
613.7'11—dc21   98-23501
CIP

First St. Martin's Griffin Edition: January 1999

3 5 7 9 10 8 6 4 2

CONTENTS

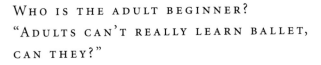
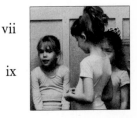
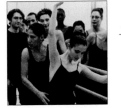
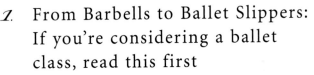
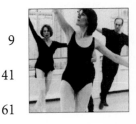
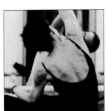
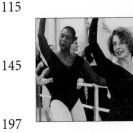

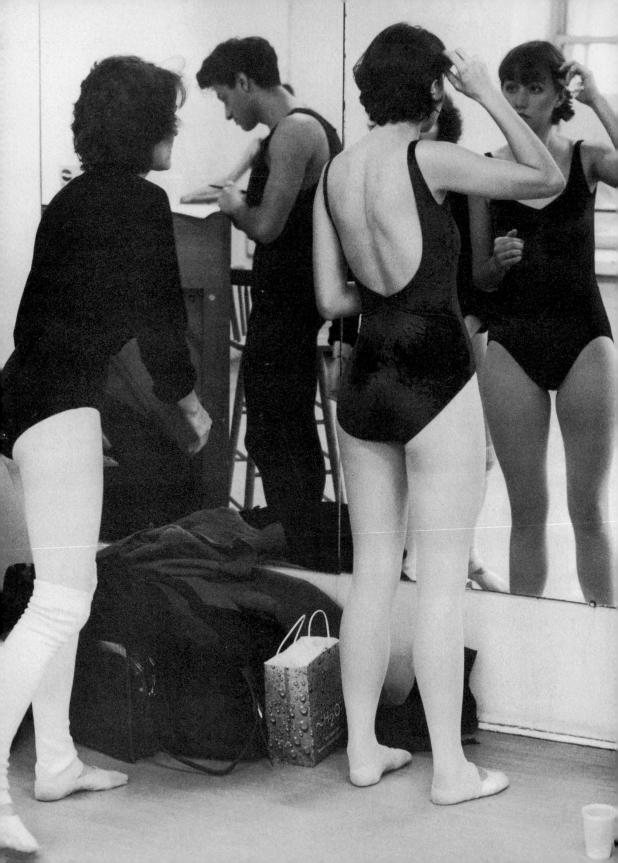

*W*ho is the adult beginner?

THIS BOOK IS FOR the adult beginner ballet student—the adult beginner of 17, the adult beginner of 70, and all of you in between. In general, by adult, we mean everyone who is introduced to the study of ballet in their teens or later, or who is returning to ballet class after a hiatus of several years, or even several decades. With a few exceptions (which we'll talk about in the pages ahead), the adult ballet beginner is not heading for a performing career but is pursuing ballet with the nonprofessional goals of fitness, relaxation, and pleasure in mind.

—DSM and AKL

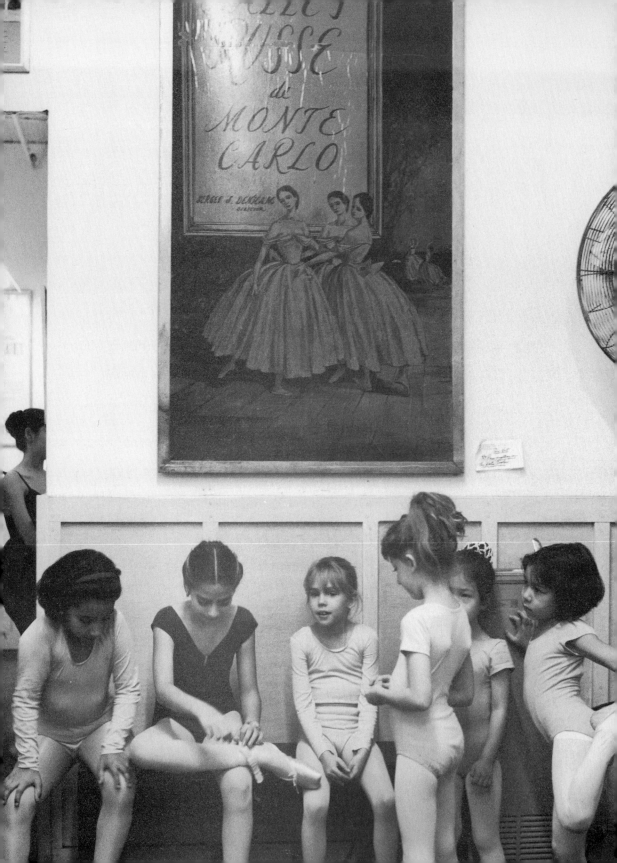

INTRODUCTION

"Adults can't really learn ballet, can they?"

❧

O H   Y E S ,   T H E Y   C A N .   In the chapters ahead, with straight talk, real-life answers, and insider's tips, we will guide you gently through the sometimes intimidating but always rewarding world of the adult ballet class.

We'll decode the steps, decipher unfamiliar vocabulary, describe the body benefits, and defuse the most common fears adults have expressed to us: "I'm uncoordinated"; "I'm not graceful"; "I've been to the ballet and my body just can't do that!" We'll spell out exactly what to expect in a typical adult beginner's class (the warm-up, the stretches, the exercises); ballet class etiquette; how to know if you're doing too much, too soon; how to avoid the most common errors; even how to dress.

As a faculty member of the Joffrey Ballet School who specializes in teaching children and adult beginners (DSM) and a writer (AKL) who is an adult ballet student, we're covering familiar and beloved territory, albeit from different directions and with different perspectives. But we are agreed that the physical benefits and emotional pleasures of ballet study at this level are well worth the effort. Plus, exercise classes based on the body-toning movements of ballet represent one of the fastest-growing segments of the fitness scene in years. What this book will give you is the information that will help you become a part of it.

In researching this book, we've sought out many experts, especially the invaluable experience that other Joffrey Ballet School faculty have had in teaching adult ballet. We've also relied on responses from nearly 500 comprehensive *Ballet-Fit* questionnaires distributed to the Joffrey Ballet School's dedicated adult beginners, to adult beginners at schools that are members of the National Association of Dance Schools, as well as to other selected dance studios and schools across the country.

Insights and comments from these questionnaires from students of all ages, backgrounds, and in different parts of the country have been helpful in determining the needs and concerns of adult ballet beginners and in assembling the *Ballet-Fit* Source Directory. This directory includes a sampling of the many ballet schools nationwide that offer nonprofessional classes; by-mail resources for ballet slippers, *pointe* shoes, clothing, and other dance paraphernalia; dance-related organizations, books, publications and CD-ROMs; plus sources for audiotapes and videotapes for the many students who have indicated a desire to practice when they're at home, traveling, or unable to attend their regular classes.

We've also interviewed other adults who are intrigued by the notion of ballet for fitness purposes but who just haven't taken the plunge. "Adults can't really learn ballet, can they?" one late thirtyish woman asked us wistfully as she watched her nine-year-old daughter practicing *pliés* in a Saturday-morning Joffrey Ballet School class. "It's something that you have to start when you're six or seven years old, isn't it?"

In fact, we found that she was voicing one of the most common misconceptions that still lingers around the ballet studio: that ballet—and, the superb workout you get with it—is for children only. In other words, no adults need apply!

To our surprise, this belief turned out to be shared by many otherwise exercise-savvy adults, in their twenties, thirties, forties, fifties, and beyond, who sweat it out in aerobics classes; play tennis and racquetball; who have mastered step and toyed with boxing—but who mistakenly believe that they're past being able to handle *pliés* and *tendus.*

We concede that if you hang around your local ballet school or dance studio, at first glance, it probably will seem to be filled with long-legged, lean-limbed adolescents, with tight little hair buns, stern little faces, and rumpled leg warmers around their ankles.

But if you look again (this time more closely) chances are the 23-year-old stretching on the floor isn't a budding ballerina but a law student who finds beginning ballet a relaxing break from her books. As for the thirty-something woman at the barre, very likely she's a new mother who's thrilled with the stronger, firmer, more flexible body she has developed since she began classes.

We want to emphasize that adult ballet beginners are a wonderful and varied group—men and women, young and old, all ages, all occupations, all levels of expertise, all degrees of physical conditioning, and with unusually diverse reasons for being there.

THE

Joffrey
Ballet School's

BALLET-FIT

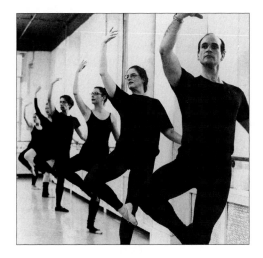

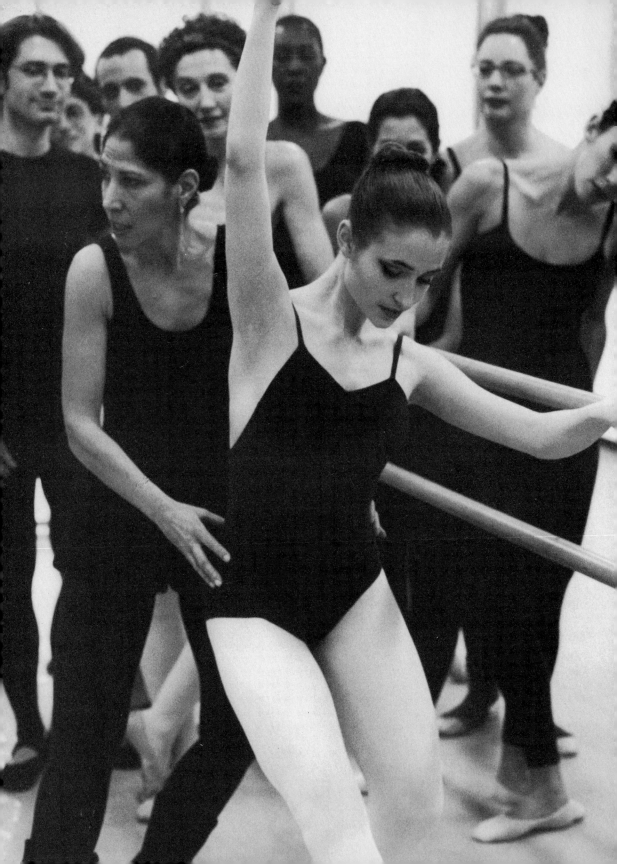

From Barbells to Ballet Slippers: If you're considering a ballet class, read this first

❧

BALLET FITNESS IS TOTAL FITNESS—body and mind—not just for your teens but for a lifetime. Overwhelmingly, as our needs and expectations from fitness have evolved, adult beginners are flocking to ballet class not just for their bodies, but for their heads. And, overwhelmingly, the ballet-fitness world is embracing adults of all ages and abilities.

The increasing number of ballet and ballet-based fitness classes represents one of the biggest shifts on the workout scene in years. Five years ago, ballet was a word you probably didn't hear often—except perhaps in elite circles. Now it seems that half the world has given up aerobics for some form of ballet-based dance.

We're not surprised by this melding of ballet and exercise, as a longer, more lithe, more fluid and feminine look—a dancer's look—has edged aside the bulkier, more muscle-bound body ideals of the last decade (fitness trends do run in cycles). It's a look that's not achieved by heavy-duty weight training (which tends to build bulky muscles) or high-impact aerobics (all those injuries) but by ballet and the body-toning movements adapted from dance.

As statistics reveal decreasing satisfaction and attendance—and a high injury rate—at overrigorous aerobic workouts (down more than 11 percent in 1995 alone according to *Health* magazine) ballet and dance have moved to the forefront. "Ballet is the perfect balance between aerobics (exercise) and yoga (soothing/focus-building) for me," writes Sarah, a 27-year-old, Boston-based graphics designer who has been attending adult ballet classes one or two times a week for about a year. "I get a bit of both in one—which is great given my tight schedule." Anna, an architect in her forties whose daughters take classes in the Joffrey Ballet School's children's division, had tried aerobics, Tai Chi, and other dance classes, but quickly gave them up. "Besides walking, it's the only exercise I get and the only thing I do just for myself. Plus, it's never too late to learn something new," she adds. For Mark, a 25-year-old performer active in regional theater, ballet is not only part of his professional training, it's fun. "I just enjoy the art—or trying to make it art," he says. "A good class makes me feel good—as if I had passed a difficult exam or taken a great vacation."

Health magazine, characterizing aerobics as "robotic and repetitive," cites boredom with the current exercise scene as a key contributing factor to the dance boom (despite the introduction of activities like slide and step). "Bored with exercise machines and tired of mechanically stepping up and down, an increasing number of women are trading in their aerobics shoes for ballet slippers, leaving the gym for traditional dance stu-

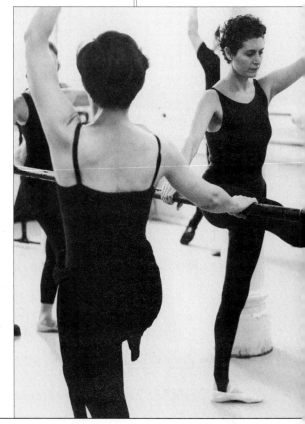

dios," *Health* magazine reports. Kathleen, 43, a New York securities analyst who studied ballet as a child and modern dance as a young adult, is one of those women turned off by gyms and what she describes as "mindless step/aerobics classes." Her initial fear of reentering a studio was quickly replaced with a sense of calm, she told us. "Ballet," she explained, "is simply a more interesting and challenging form of exercise."

The feelings expressed by Sarah, Anna, Mark, and Kathleen are representative of thousands of men and women across the country, as seen by the increasing number of fitness classes cropping up at health clubs, spas, and fitness centers that borrow the movements of classical ballet training. In fact, many experts believe that soon virtually all gyms will be offering dance or movement-based classes for its members.

At the ballet schools themselves, nonprofessional enrollment, particularly for adults over 35, is on the upswing (it's the fastest growing segment of the dance world). *Dance* magazine cites a recent Mellon Foundation survey of ballet schools nationwide, which finds that more than 75 percent of ballet schools now offer nonprofessional adult classes. On the average, adult students (again, on the nonprofessional level) constitute nearly half of these schools' enrollment.

And it's small wonder. As ballet star Allegra Kent points out in *The Dancer's Body Book,* ballet dancers have the strongest, most beautiful, and very probably the most envied bodies in the world. When properly executed, ballet movements sculpt muscles so that they become taut, lean, and beautiful. "During the last year, coming to class two to three times a week, I've noticed a lengthening of muscles, particularly the legs, and a reshaping of [my] hips and buttocks," reports one Joffrey Ballet School adult beginner. Other students from all over the country collectively report firmer abdominal muscles, stronger legs, and more shapely thighs. "I now have dancer's calves," marvels Leslie, a 41-year-old attorney, who seldom misses her twice-weekly classes. "And my whole body is much stronger."

Many of the Joffrey Ballet School adult ballet beginners surveyed attend ballet classes two and three times a week. But even those who barely manage a single class see a difference in their bodies in a relatively short time. (Getting to class doesn't take extra time, just the wise use of the time you have!) As one student put it: "Throughout the day, I find myself practicing steps while waiting in the elevator, standing on line, or in my office. I have wanted to take formal lessons for a while; I'm so glad I made the time."

More Than a Workout

Before we get into any of the ballet class specifics, there is an important point that we want to make: Many different forms of exercise work. The trick is finding the one that's right for you, meaning not just one you're likely to stick with but one that you'll enjoy.

And that's where you'll find that adult ballet more than holds its own. Ballet appeals to jaded exercisers because it's much more than a workout; it's pleasurable in a way that using a StairMaster or treadmill three times a week simply isn't. "I am much more motivated to take a ballet class than I am to go to the gym for a more conventional workout," concurs Jennifer, 29, a graduate student in literature who alternates twice-weekly ballet classes with flamenco lessons. "In fact, dance classes are now my primary means of exercise."

Adults tend to take to ballet class because even the simplest movements at the barre can be expressive and because ballet class provides an intellectual element along with the physical. "Ballet is beautiful because it works. I love how all the moves are integral and flow together to form a dance," explains Kasey, a 21-year-old beginner from Philadelphia who began classes as a college senior. "We respond in a visceral and emotional sense, as much as a physical one," points out Lianna, a 35-year-old Chicago mother of two who fondly remembers her childhood classes and early exploits *en pointe.* (For parents who have children currently in ballet classes, adult ballet offers a special method of communication and bonding. "It's something my daughter and I share," explains another ballet mom, also from Chicago, who fills the time her 10-year-old is in ballet class by taking her own ballet stretch class. "Plus now I know a lot more about what she's doing.")

Consistently, the adult students surveyed cite the emotional satisfactions of ballet class, as much as they do the physical ones. "I'm completely relaxed by the end of class—all the cobwebs are cleared out of my brain," confesses Claire, a New York advertising executive in her forties who had taken ballet class as a child and in her early thirties. "The concentration needed for ballet means that any worries and problems are forced out of the brain for the duration of class," points out Amanda, a 56-year-old homemaker from Maryland who has been taking twice-weekly classes for 17 years. "And the good feeling usually lingers," she adds. Tony, a 30-year-old

At the end of class, students get a chance to dance across the floor.

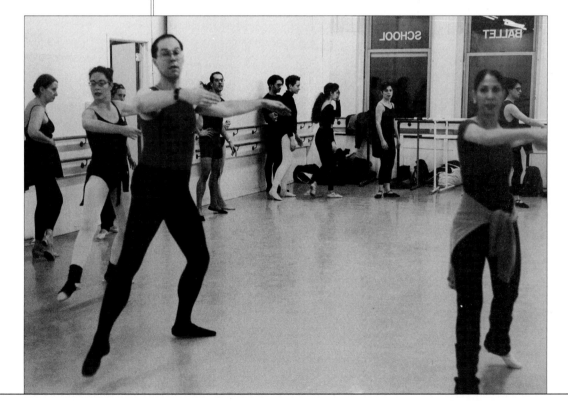

financial analyst who takes class at the Joffrey Ballet School, also finds that the intense focus and concentrated effort of his class serve as both an emotional and psychological release. As for Britt, a 37-year-old actress and mother, also a Joffrey adult beginner, she finds that not only has ballet class made her more confident, but emotionally stronger to negotiate with her children and their lives.

"Benefits" like these might not be expected, but they are a welcome bonus—and a significant part of the total package that your ballet class may deliver (for some people, when all is said and done, it might just be its biggest justification). Many adult students find ballet class in the words of one survey participant, "a welcome antidote to work." "Dancing provides a complete change of focus for me," says Carol, a 49-year-old book editor. "Spatially, from close concentration to an emphasis on using space; psychologically, by going from being the boss to being a student; emotionally, by 'exposing' myself and being with others; physically, by having to

Ballet students of all ages learn basic positions at the barre. Here, sous-sus, *with arms* en haut.

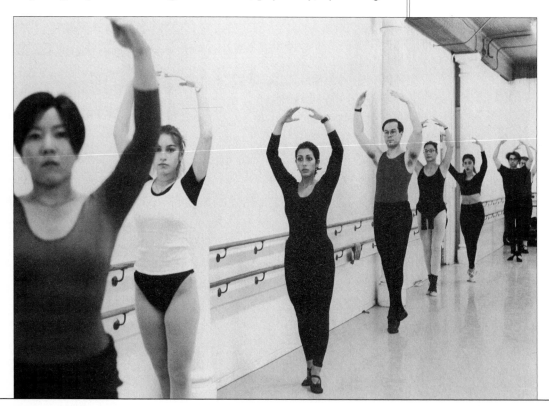

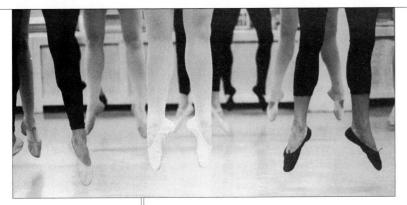

Feet need time to learn to point. Adult feet vary in their flexibility and strength. Little jumps (sautés) in first position help strengthen the feet.

work hard and get stronger." Concludes another student: "It's the ultimate in stress relief. It's almost as good as a massage—and it's much cheaper than a therapist!"

Finally, taking it all one step further, ballet, unlike more mundane forms of exercise, has the uncanny power to inspire deep passion and fealty among its devotees. "I am happier and calmer because I am doing what I love the most," writes a 51-year-old New York artist (who also notes that you don't get good posture from a StairMaster!). "In the words of Joseph Campbell, I am following my bliss. It is my soul." Admits 26-year-old Sabrina, a computer specialist who does a full half-hour barre every day: "I love it! I love it! I love it! When I have a good class, I feel like I can fly. Nothing makes me happier." Lynn, also in her twenties, says that studying ballet today is more rewarding than it was when she was 12, when she seriously longed for a dance career. "Now it's about learning for the sake of learning, not because I may someday be a famous ballerina. Although," she adds with a wink, "you never know . . ."

It's in response to all the adults all over the country who are taking up the challenge of ballet—and especially to all the beautiful and inspiring Joffrey Ballet School adult beginners—that we've put together this book: a realistic guide to learning ballet, with lifelong fitness in mind, even though you're all grown up.

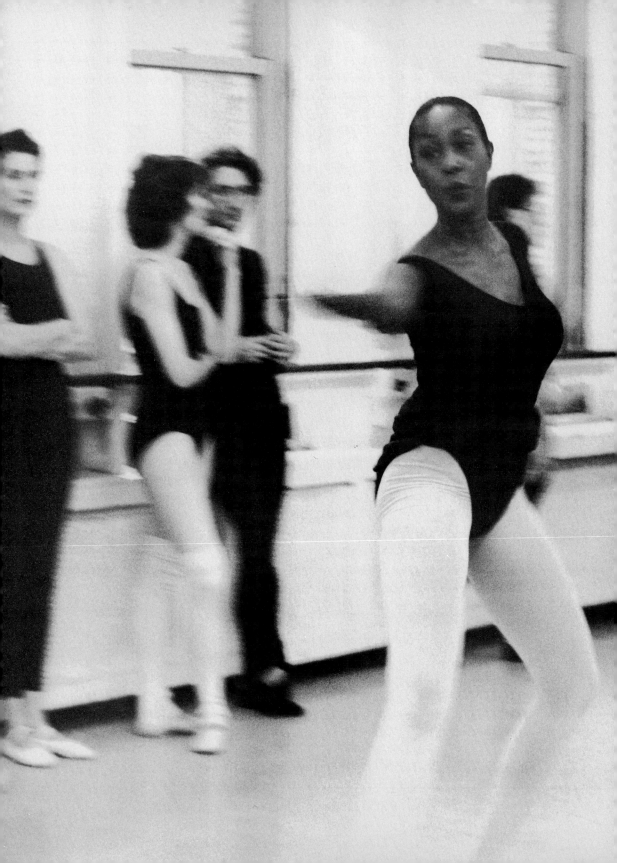

2

$\mathcal{S}$ tarting Out:
What to expect . . .
and why

IT'S TRADITION

THIS IS WHERE IT STARTS, the how-tos of finding the adult ballet class you've been reading about and, we hope, looking forward to. The good news is that when you walk into any ballet school or studio, anywhere in the country, the class you'll experience will be essentially the same. In a ballet school in Hartford, or a dance studio in San Diego, or in Minneapolis or Houston—or at the Joffrey Ballet School in New York City—each class begins with *pliés* at the barre (sometimes preceded by a series of simple limbering stretches and bends). Then, it moves into *tendu* exercises to warm up the foot, then *dégagés* and *ronds des jambes* (on the floor and off—keep that heel forward—yes, it is hard!). On to *frappés,* the anomaly at the barre (the only exercise that calls for a flexed foot, it's the bane of many an adult beginner's existence). Next, an *adagio*—that's a slow stretch at the barre, usually incorporating *développés, fondus,* and other movements—followed by *grands battements,* an exuberant leg stretch, lifting the leg high.

After the barre, the Joffrey Ballet School and many ballet schools and studios (though not all), offer floor exercises to further strengthen the muscles. These also help illustrate correct placement, without the burden of balancing the weight of the body at the same time. If there are men in the class, push-ups may be added. (Yes, we know it's sexist, but theoretically, male performers do have to lift and carry their female partners. In the *Ballet-Fit* Workout [see page 145], we've given the option of a modified women's push-up, should any of you be so moved.)

The third and final portion of the class is known as "center"; its actual components are at the teacher's discretion. A typical center has four distinct parts:

1. *adagio* steps, including turns and preparations for turns that start out simple but gradually become more difficult, often with head and arm movements added;
2. *petit allegro,* which means small jumps like *changements;*
3. *grand allegro,* which calls for bigger combinations on the diagonal (these are what get you really moving); and
4. a cool-down, which might include *grands battements* (high kicks) or perhaps *port de bras* (graceful arm movements).

All of these, of course, are performed in the center of the studio without the aid of the barre.

Even as the ballet class moves to a more advanced level, there's little change from the familiar sequence of combinations we've described above (which, you'll notice, begins with small leg movements that gradually become bigger, higher, and faster, as the body warms up and the leg is lifted from the floor). The tempo quickens; combinations of steps become longer and more complex, but except for minor variations, based on your teacher's style, taste, and whim, the pattern is already set. Wherever you live, wherever you travel, wherever you take a class, you can rely on the classic movements to be essentially the same.

And for good reason: The traditional ballet workout does indeed work. It has for centuries.

Ballet is part of a tradition that developed in 17th-century France in the court of the Sun King, Louis XIV, but its roots go back even further. The movements you learn in the local ballet class in your hometown (the concept of turnout, the five positions of the feet) are based on those that developed at the very first ballet school, L'Académie Royale de la Danse, which was founded in 1661. (This explains why, to this day, French—of sorts—is the language of ballet.) And the movements have undergone no radical changes since. Instead, there's been an evolution: from court dancing, huge costumes, and male-only dancers to *pointe* work, light costumes, and female dancers, to Russian and Neo-Classical modes and almost no costumes at all!

Standing at the barre, the class has feet in first, arms à la seconde.

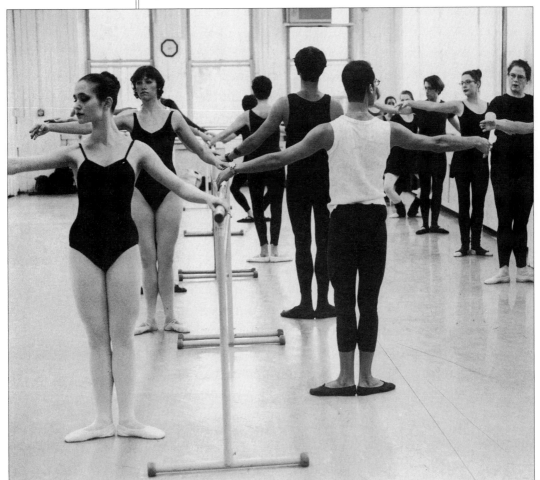

Since that time, each ballet teacher has passed on what he or she knows, continuing hundreds of years of ballet tradition. Why, for example, do most teachers start class with the right side, left hand on the barre? Because it's ballet tradition. It's always been done that way.

Of course, to today's sophisticated dance audiences, the first ballet performances would hardly be recognized as such. In fact, the earliest ballets were court ballets—highly stylized, ceremonial stories, told through movement, dialogue and song, and featuring many of the stock characters of the *commedia dell'arte* tradition. It wasn't until the 18th century that dialogue gradually disappeared and stories began to be told exclusively through dance, which was gaining recognition as an art form in and of itself.

It was the 19th century that saw the beginnings of ballet as we know it today, when the same romanticism that manifested itself in literature, poetry, and the fine and decorative arts had its effect on dance. Blocked shoes were invented, and for the first time, female dancers appeared *en pointe.* The great Romantic ballets of the 1830s *(La Sylphide, Giselle)* were created, and with the introduction of new, filmy, calf-length skirts, the illusion of the ballet dancer as a weightless, ethereal, utterly romantic creature was complete. Soon, the cult of the ballerina was born with female stars such as Maria Taglioni (the archetypal Romantic ballerina) and her earthier rival, Fanny Elssler, who were worshiped and idealized, much as Hollywood stars are today.

Even as the roots of ballet tradition extend back to Europe, in the 20th century, ballet's most fertile branches have been decidedly American. Robert Joffrey, an ambitious young dancer hailing from Seattle, was the first classical choreographer who didn't look back to Europe for inspiration but whose goal was to create an indigenous American ballet. In making his name, Joffrey, who died in 1988, created a uniquely American ballet school to train dancers for what would become a uniquely American company.

In 1952, with his friend and colleague Gerald Arpino, Joffrey founded what is formally known as the Joffrey Ballet School–

If you're looking for self-expression or spontaneity of movement in your adult beginner ballet class, you're going to be disappointed. As you'll see in the pages ahead, ballet exercises at the barre or even in the center leave little room for innovation (accept it: these days, there are few, if any, classics around). In consolation, let us explain that a specific and deliberate purpose underscores every step, every gesture, and every ballet movement: to warm, strengthen, and lengthen particular muscles for the physical demands of the dance.

American Ballet Center to develop and train professional dancers. Four years later, Robert Joffrey's Theater Dancers (later the City Center Joffrey Ballet; now the Joffrey Ballet of Chicago) made its first tour. It's through these two venues, his New York training school and his company, that Joffrey is credited by many as having brought ballet to the popular consciousness of the American public.

Today, students of the Joffrey Ballet School, located in New York City, "graduate" not only to the Joffrey Ballet Company but to companies all over the United States, Canada, and throughout Europe.

So there's profound ritual involved. And history. And it is this long, honored, and rather glamorous tradition that sets ballet apart from the aerobics class at your local gym or calisthenics at the Y. Ballet is more than a sport; it's an art. Moreover, it's the ephemeral art of Pavlova, Marius Petipa, Fokine and Diaghilev, Nijinsky, Balanchine, Robert Joffrey, and other modern-day luminaries, with an underlying mystique that remains intact to this day.

Sometimes subconsciously (although, we have to admit, sometimes deliberately too), dancers, dance teachers, and even dance students conspire to preserve and protect this precious mystique (believe us, the chill that many newcomers feel on entering the dance studio can be very real—and it has nothing to do with faulty air conditioning!). This cultivated mystique is what sets dancers apart from ordinary, earthbound mortals, and it's what makes the ballet world so forbidding—at first—to adult beginners. "Often good schools don't take adult classes seriously," laments a 36-year-old dance videographer in Hartford, Connecticut, who has been taking ballet class since she was six. "They should, if only as dance audience development." Another adult student in Washington, D.C., now in her late thirties, credits her good luck in finding an adults-only ballet studio that "was serious, but without pretensions or competitiveness on the part of the faculty or students" for getting her "restarted" on ballet eleven years ago.

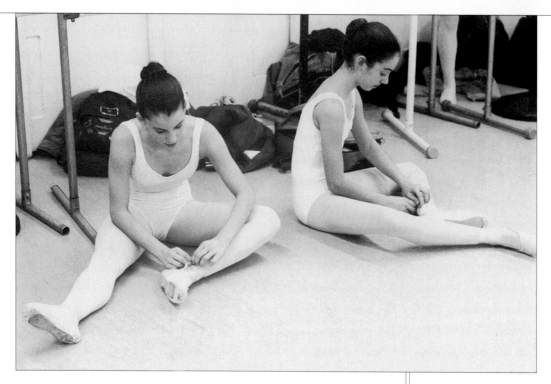

To be fair, insider "clubbiness" exists in every profession. In the dance world, however, perhaps outsiders tend to feel it a little more personally because competence rests on physical prowess and because of ballet's regal history. After all, ballet *was* originally performed for kings and emperors!

Expect to see serious young students at your school or studio, but don't let them intimidate you.

EXPLODING THE MYTHS

Like opera, classical music, and other so-called higher arts, the ballet world is enwrapped in the aura of culture, an art only appreciated by the educated and executed by the physical elite. Its practice is for the select few, and many of its rituals tend to sustain that notion. Indeed, often adult beginners are discouraged from even attempting ballet. Alas, we're told, there are certain things that only the young can learn. As for adult *pointe* work, the party line says it's a near-abomination—not to mention downright dangerous.

Beliefs like these represent lingering bits of ballet myth to which no one should be subscribing in the 1990s and beyond (besides, it's in the interest of dancers to encourage a more involved, more knowledgeable audience). Still, what this picture should tell you—and fast—is that you're going to have to keep your own needs, demands—and limitations—firmly in mind.

For the record: We feel that efforts to discourage adults from taking appropriate ballet classes are unfortunate. These efforts seem to be widely perpetuated both by teachers who have had performing careers and those who haven't, who seem to join in a sometimes unconscious effort to make adult beginners uncomfortable about even considering stretching their legs into *arabesque,* let alone attempting their first wobbly *pirouettes!*

The fact is, nonperforming dance instructors may be, at heart, frustrated performers, while former dancers may think they're beyond teaching adults (or children, for that matter). But it's the gifted teacher who can instill in these groups a love and passion for the art. Plus, as one canny dance educator noted to us, it doesn't take much to teach a corps of talented, motivated, advanced intermediates!

Adults can be serious students also, even if they don't aspire to perform.

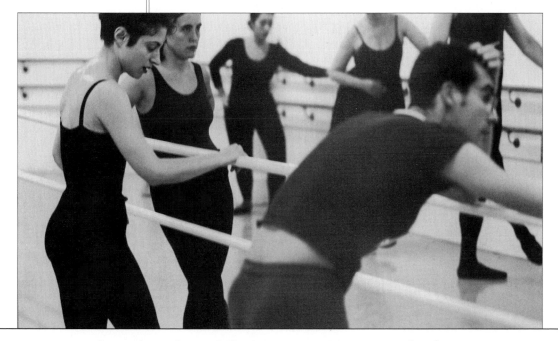

Well, we're here to open the doors. To explode the myths and correct the misconceptions. To welcome you, the adult beginner—warmly—to the world of ballet fitness. The reality is that while not everyone can dance at a performance level on the stage, anyone can learn ballet, especially the body-toning, muscle-strengthening barre and floor exercises. Anyone can learn them and any body can benefit from their physical and emotional benefits.

So, let's begin.

FIFTEEN BALLET FEARS AND HOW TO GET PAST THEM

It starts inside your head. The hesitation. The uncertainty. And discomfiture—perhaps about your age, perhaps about your body, perhaps about your ability (after all, you don't want to put yourself in a position where you're going to look—and feel—foolish). And it's this kind of thinking that's a trap.

Trust us: We do understand. The fact is, ballet studios are intimidating. There's that gorgeous girl at the desk. And all those skinny students. What so many adults tend to forget is that everyone feels the same way at first. So let's address, and hopefully dispel, the fifteen most common ballet fears that hold back so many people.

1. "I'd feel out of place. I don't want to be in a class with a bunch of kids or with professional dancers who will make me feel foolish."

Go back and reread the introduction to this book. As we've explained, ballet students come in all ages, sexes, shapes, and sizes! Plus, good old common sense should tell you that professionals, or anyone training to be, will not be taking an adult beginner class! A once-in-a-while exception: When a professional wants to work at a slower pace (when they're recovering from an injury or perhaps attached to a particular teacher's method). But don't be intimidated. Any professional in a beginner class is there for his or her own

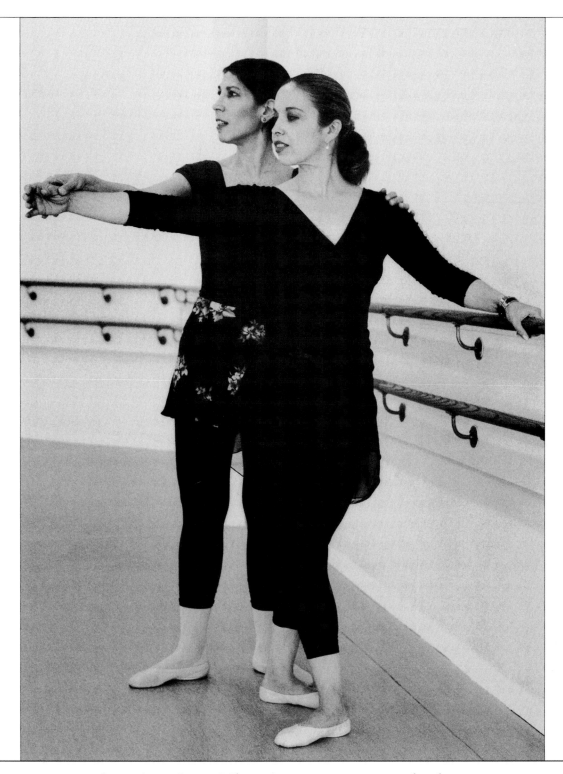

reasons, which don't include looking at you! We have it on good authority that professionals have a ton of respect for adult beginners. After all, who knows better just how demanding ballet really is? Besides, your desire to try it is a great compliment to them!

2. "I've been to the ballet. I could never do what they do."

Absolutely true! Dancers training for a professional career spend their entire lives preparing their bodies for dance, and usually take at least two classes a day in order to do what they do. Performing professionals generally take a company class in the morning, rehearse all day, and perform at night. But an adult beginner class isn't a performance; you're not going to do what they do. Look at it this way: As an adult, you can draw on skills, talents, and experiences ballet dancers don't have. Use them to enhance your deeper understanding of the art.

3. "Dancers are thin; I'm too fat. I'll have to show up in one of those skimpy leotards that show everything."

We said all sizes, that means size 4, size 14, whatever. One regular in our adult beginner classes is a 60-year-old former professional dancer, now a professor of theater and speech. At five feet five inches and 145 pounds, she asked us to please deal with the myth that you have to be barely 100 pounds to dance ballet. If you're more comfortable, cover up with a T-shirt. A sweatshirt. Sweatpants, leggings, shorts, or a wisp of a dance skirt (although we do think some of these skirts provide more psychological coverage than anything else). Once you become a regular (and feel more at ease), you'll probably start to shed layers (and possibly a few pounds). For more about the ins and outs of what to wear, see chapter 4.

4. "I'm uncoordinated (I could never even learn to play tennis). And I'm not flexible. I can't do a split."

Okay, coordination helps, but joining an adult ballet class isn't like trying out for the Rockettes! Besides, you learn coordination (that's why you're in a beginner class). If you're not flexible to start, that will improve too. As for splits, stop worrying. No adult ballet class we've ever visited requires its students to execute a split.

5. "I'm not musical. I just don't get how the music relates to the movement."

We hear this a lot. But you may be more musical than you think: Movement to music is almost instinctive. Besides, many terrific dance students are near musical illiterates. But it doesn't mean that they don't feel the music in class. Plus, we *teach* music in class.

6. "I'm not graceful. Never was, never could be. And I can't dance on my toes."

No adult beginner is—at first. Give it time. And, believe it or not, offstage, often professional dancers tend to be clumsy (like swans out of water, so to speak). As for working *en pointe,* that's not what ballet fitness is all about, nor is it realistic for most adults. Adult beginner classes are taken in regular flat ballet slippers.

For the dedicated adult student who wants to make *pointe* a goal, it's a valid and exciting one, but it is long-range. For those adult students who are able to develop their strength and technique to the level where they can capably start *pointe* work, see Chapter 8.

7. "Ballet is expensive. I'll have to buy all new clothes and shoes."

Compared to the cost of a gym membership (which you may hardly ever use), an adult ballet class could very well be the fitness bargain of your life. Plus, ballet classes show up in many unlikely places, from your local Y to your high school's adult-education center, so be sure to explore all your options. New clothes? We're not talking designer tutus! Go shopping in your own closet and you'll probably find appropriate clothes for ballet class and won't even have to think about anything new. Ballet shoes are a necessity, though, but they cost a whole lot less than Reeboks, RollerBlades, or ski boots. Plan on spending about $12 to $15 for canvas ballet shoes, about $25 to $28 for leather ones.

8. "There isn't any place to study where I live."

That's where the *Ballet-Fit* Source Directory comes in. Use it to track down the class nearest you or to send for an at-home ballet video or audiotape. Or consider starting a class with interested friends.

9. "I don't have the look. I can't put my hair up in a bun."

Okay, we admit there is a stereotypical ballet "look": long legs, small head, flexible body. But it's a look—an illusion—and one you might have too, someday (it's really the look of being fit, healthy, and confident). Your hair? Just get it out of your eyes.

10. "I'd be embarrassed. I don't want to be laughed at when I make a mistake."

Some adults report to us that one of the most satisfying things about ballet class is the anonymity: Students are so focused on what they're doing (there is a lot to remember!) that no one is looking at anyone else. Invariably, students concentrate on themselves in the mirror, constantly checking to see that their hips are square, their shoulders down, their heels forward. You set the standard; you and you alone are your own measure of progress.

11. "Ballet is too rigid and structured for my personality."

There *is* a structure to ballet, but the fact is that structure is the basis of every other form of dance. Besides, it's only an hour and a half or so out of your life—surely, every life can deal with that much structure! Plus, many people, even the most high-powered types, find comfort and relaxation in giving up the decision-making process for an hour or so, and not having to think about what comes next.

12. **"Ballet is a girlie-girl kind of thing. I'm beyond that."**

What can we say? Tell that to some of the guys in the class and watch a few necks bristle. You may think of ballet as pink tulle and satin, but there are plenty of runners, weight lifters, and Tai Chi masters lining up at the barre. Vince Lombardi, the *very* macho coach of the legendary Green Bay Packers, had his players take ballet—for coordination, discipline, and endurance.

13. **"All the steps are in French and I don't speak French. I won't know what the teacher is talking about."**

You may not be able to understand your teacher, but it won't be because he or she is speaking French! Ballet classes are in English, even though the steps have French names (see Chapter 5, "The Language of Ballet"). Plus, it's not French—it's ballet French (which is fractured at best!).

14. **"I can't concentrate. I would never be able to remember all those sequences."**

This happens. A lot. Especially to working adults coming straight from the office. Most teachers understand this. In some cases, the teacher may be giving combinations that are too long and complex (combinations should be short, logical, and appropriate to a beginner level). But if the combinations are sensible, try strategic positioning behind a more experienced student whom you can follow easily. And hang in there. Through familiarity and repetition, repetition, repetition, the muscles eventually remember.

15. **"I have a lot of physical problems—old sports injuries, bad knees . . ."**

Everyone who is interested should try an adult beginner class. If you have problems with your knees or with your back, you may need to modify or eliminate certain movements. On the other hand, ballet is terrific for strengthening the abdominal muscles (which help support the back), for overall muscle toning, improving flexibility, coordination, and posture. Still, always talk to your doctor first about any physical problems you may have.

SCHOOLS VERSUS STUDIOS

Throughout this text we're going to refer to ballet schools and ballet studios interchangeably. This is for our convenience, but you should know that there are differences (some of which you may care about it; some not at all).

The condensed version: A ballet school, like the Joffrey Ballet School, offers graded classes. By this we mean that classes are given on formalized levels—beginner, advanced beginner, intermediate, and so on, all supervised by a central administration. A studio, which may be less strictly monitored than a school, generally refers to an individual or group of individuals who rent space to conduct ballet classes. (Another difference, which usually matters very little to the student, is merely a matter of administrative organization. Since many schools are nonprofit and few are tuition-driven, they're frequently organized like educational institutions so they can qualify for grants.)

Should the adult beginner attend a school or a studio class? It all depends. Both, in fact, are viable options for the adult beginner. In some cases, adult beginners may be more welcome at a studio, as opposed to a school where the focus is on training professionals (which, as one Joffrey faculty member pointed out, tends to have more cachet in the ballet world). But again, it all depends on the adult, the school or studio, and the teachers' respective attitudes toward the art of teaching.

FINDING A CLASS

Sometimes, of course, it's quite clear which ballet class you're going to attend—if you live in a rural area or small town, it may be the only one for miles around! But if you have a choice—and in major

QUESTIONS TO ASK

Start your search for an appropriate class by making phone calls and asking questions.

- Is the school or studio only training dancers starting from childhood or are nonprofessional classes offered? If so, how are they graded? Can you enter an adult beginner class at any point (these are sometimes called "drop-in" classes) or do you have to start at the beginning of the term?
- When are the adult classes scheduled? Note: Be realistic about this. Can you leave your office in time to make a 6:00 P.M. class? If you take an evening class that ends at 8:30, will you miss the last train home—and will the teacher mind letting you leave 15 minutes early? Maybe there's a class on Saturday morn-

ings before you have to start in on family obligations.

- ◆ How is payment for class made? Do you have to sign up for a whole term, in which case, if you miss a class, are there make-ups? Or, as at the Joffrey Ballet School, can adults pay as they go? Ask, too, if a class card is offered, which entitles you to attend a certain number of classes, at your convenience, and at a discount (class cards sometimes entitle you to discounts on dancewear, so be sure to ask if there's a discount policy with any local merchants). If a class card is offered, is it restricted or open-ended: If you purchase, say, 15 classes but don't manage to attend them all within three months, do you forfeit the unused portion of your payment?

cities and university towns, you'll find a wealth of options—we advise observing classes at as many different schools and studios as you can.

What you're looking for, of course, is an environment that's welcoming to the adult beginner, and that may require some searching. Matthew, a 25-year-old dance student from Virginia who was introduced to ballet in college and wanted to continue, found that at many of the studios he visited, adult classes were merely an afterthought to the children's and professional classes and were treated somewhat disparagingly. "The instructors glossed over the adult students," he said, noting that "it's nice to be recognized as someone who strives to improve, even though you've started later in life." So recognize it: Some teachers just don't like teaching adults.

In looking for the right school, be prepared for trade-offs. Regina, a Washington, D.C.–based adult beginner in her thirties, was looking for a school close to her home; she was nursing an infant and couldn't afford extensive travel time. But she settled for a school a little farther away than she intended because she considered its supportive atmosphere well worth the minor inconvenience. "I stayed because of the helpful, knowledgeable, and inspiring faculty and the friendly atmosphere," she explains. She also appreciates the fact that adult students are encouraged to progress at their own pace.

WHAT'S A "BEGINNER" CLASS?

It's important to understand the integrity of the level of the class you are considering. A question to consider: If, for example, a class is described as a beginner class, is the teacher teaching it at a true beginner level? This means simple combinations, slow tempos, and plenty of verbal explanation. Adult beginner classes should not be intimidating.

In addition, you, the student, should be willing to participate

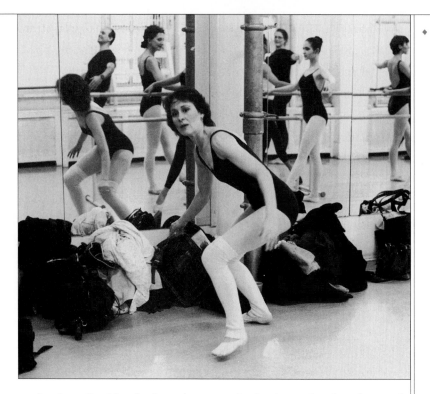

at the described level. If you are past the beginner level and attend a beginner class, don't affect a bored expression when the pace is too slow for you, or yawn as the instructor talks the class through their first *frappés*.

Integrity of levels also means that the instructor tries to move students out of the beginner class as they progress. If a student clearly is past the beginner stage, the responsible teacher has an obligation to encourage the student to take a faster class rather than adjust the level of the class to the detriment of the true beginners. In other words, if you want to work at another level, take another level.

Of course, there are legitimate instances when an experienced student might want and need the more nurturing pace of a beginner class; i.e., when recovering from an injury and needing to work slowly, when warming up for another class, or especially when working more deliberately in order to perfect a particular movement or step.

◆ Where do students leave their coats, handbags, clothes, and street shoes during class? On hooks in the dressing room? In cubbies or lockers? Do you need to bring a lock? It's not a good idea to leave anything out in a ballet school's dressing room—anywhere, even at the Joffrey Ballet School. Unless there are locked lockers, students usually bring their personal belongings into the classroom itself, and heap them in one corner, away from the door (usually near the piano).

◆ When you visit, scrutinize the facility closely, but bear in mind that ballet schools and studios are seldom as pristine and gleaming as the health club or gym you may be used to. Chances are, it has been there a long time and the emphasis is not on looks but on tradition. The Joffrey Ballet School, for example, is located in Greenwich Village's historic district, a landmark area where few architectural modernizations are permitted.

Often studio schools will be found in or near a city's theater district, and they have a tradition and look of their own. In fact, in some ways, a certain theatrical seediness is even a point of perverse pride. In a gym, if the equipment is old and rusty, it's not going to work. But all a dancer needs is a barre and a mirror in an empty space; it doesn't matter if the floor is worn or the windows not quite clean.

Many adult beginners taking ballet for fitness and relaxation purposes simply enjoy the nonpressured pace or become attached to a particular teacher and that teacher's methods, and don't care to move on. This is perfectly acceptable, too, as long as they are satisfied to continue at the level of the class. At the Joffrey Ballet School—as at most others—the teachers share their pointers on teaching and technique, but every teacher tends to have his or her own following.

Experienced adult students (let's call them advanced beginners) who are comfortable with the teacher's methods and barre are often an asset in a class, standing at either end of the barre (and placed strategically in the middle), so less secure or less experienced students can follow . . . and be inspired!

CHOOSING A TEACHER

After you find a school or studio, it's up to you to find a teacher who is simpatico. And it's only by observing and experiencing different teaching methods that you can assess the teacher or teachers to whom you'll respond best. One thing you should understand from the start is that the typical ballet class is most emphatically not a democracy! Your teacher—regardless of his or her personal style—is, by tradition, an absolute figure in the classroom (which we'll be discussing throughout this book).

At the same time, personal styles vary. Ballet teachers can be nurturing and helpful or distant and matter-of-fact. Some may carefully mark the steps with you; others may demonstrate and leave you to follow on your own. So, we stress, of course, there is no right or wrong style. What works for one person doesn't work for another.

Be honest with yourself about the role you want your teacher to play. Ballet teachers often find themselves thrust into a variety of roles that go beyond the required job of effectively teaching the class. Often they're privy to personal confidences and confessions, which may not always be appropriate. So search your soul a bit here. Are you looking for a mommy, a new best friend, a shrink, a career counselor, a diet buddy? Or (we hope) simply a terrific and satisfying new way to stay fit?

At the same time, your relationship with your teacher is a two-way street, so consider your teacher's attitude as well. His or her frustrations are not your business and shouldn't get in the way of your learning (which will happen only if you allow it). In our experience, most ballet teachers have something wonderful to offer; it's up to you to accept it. And the only way you're going to learn is by taking that first step—and first class.

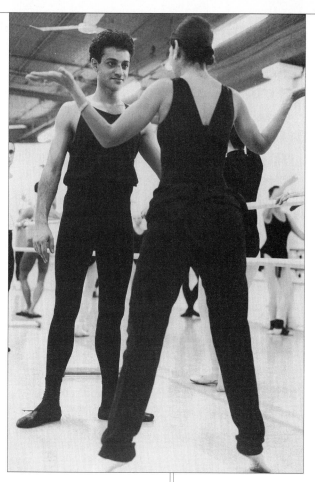

Individual corrections create rapport between teacher and students, and benefit the whole class as well. Here, Sasha learns how to balance on two feet en relevé.

REMEMBER: BALLET *IS* A PERFORMING ART

Even though you're studying ballet for fitness and pleasure, keep in mind that you are learning a performing art, an art intended for an audience. It's for this reason that many teachers make special efforts to distance the atmosphere of the ballet class from that of the gym, even to the point of discouraging students from wearing gym-oriented workout wear.

Even though you are not there for performance training, the fact that ballet is a performing art may very well affect the "tone" of the class to a greater or lesser degree depending on your individual teacher.

Zelma Bustillo, a former member of the Joffrey Ballet Company who now teaches at the Joffrey School, points out that understanding the motivations of her adult students was a turning point for her as a teacher. "Years ago, I wondered why adults would want to do ballet, instead of aerobics or gymnastics, which are certainly effective fitness techniques," she remembers. "But once I saw that the adults loved and were inspired by ballet in the same way that I am—they just were coming to it at a later date and with other considerations—it made a huge difference."

In a professional company, Bustillo explains, you are reprimanded if you miss a class. "But adults who come to class don't have that external pressure; the commitment to come to class is within themselves," she points out. "Realizing that inspired me and made me enjoy teaching adults because they truly care and make the effort to be there."

Frequently, for example, teachers may make allusions to how a certain step is performed on stage or tell a class to present their heels to "the audience" (which is the mirror). This is simply part of the professional atmosphere of the class. It's not meant to be patronizing, nor is it an invitation to indulge in ballerina fantasies on the part of otherwise sensible adults.

Instead, take the teacher's occasional references to the stage in the spirit in which they are given. "It has to do with the reality of what you are doing, which is something many adults don't necessarily think about at first," explains Sidney Lowenthal, who is a former performer and a member of the Joffrey Ballet School's faculty, with many years of experience in teaching adults. "Adults may come in at first for the exercise or the music—or for a combination of both—but there's more to it than that." For example, in explaining the history of ballet and its origins in the courts of France, Lowenthal might urge her adults to repeat a series of steps as if they were doing them for the French king. Or to imagine themselves on stage at the Met. "It's a fantasy and a few eyes do roll," she admits, "and, of course, you've got to do it with humor. Still, for that moment in time for the students who go along with it, I see their movements become bigger and more true."

"The minute you walk into a studio, and there is a mirror and music and other people—even if they are just other students in the class—it is a performance, though, of course, not in the professional sense," insists Andrei Kulyk, another Joffrey Ballet School teacher who started performing as a child. "While, in a sense, we are duplicating a stage situation, the classroom is the safest stage there is," he adds. "In fact, it's risk-free. No one is going to throw vegetables at you or ask for their ticket money back."

Kulyk feels, as do other teachers across the country, that it benefits the adult to think in terms of performance because it enhances the whole ballet experience. "Even though there are introverts and extroverts—and performers and nonperformers—I personally believe that inside every single person there is a performer, because

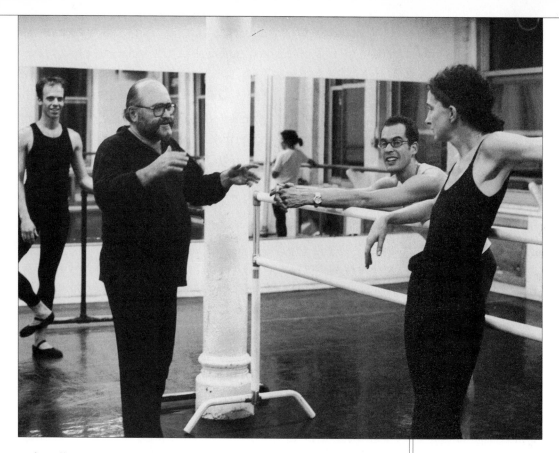

we're all social creatures—and, in life, we perform all the time. In ballet class, it's just a matter of taking that extra step."

At the same time, it's also understood that references to the "audience" and performance-oriented corrections are not intended to prepare adult students to perform but are part of the technique of teaching a performing art.

At the Joffrey School, Andrei Kulyk prefers general corrections, and his class seems to enjoy them.

CONSIDERING THE ADULT CLASS (NOW YOU ARE SIX . . . AGAIN!)

The adult ballet beginner—of any age—should realize that ballet can be a bit infantilizing: It's the nature of the process. As a ballet student, you are putting yourself in the hands of a parental figure and expected to follow directions largely without dialogue, without

TAKING A PROFESSIONAL CLASS

The adult beginner who inadvertently wanders into a professional class will stick out like a sore thumb, by virtue of age, often shape, and level of competence. But what if there simply are no other adult classes in your area?

If you have no alternative, observe the class carefully before you attend and talk frankly with the teacher to determine your comfort level. Even if the teacher tells you that he or she doesn't mind if you take the class, you may not get the attention you are looking for (and in some cases, the attention may be negative!).

If your ego can handle it, stay in the back; take the class for what it's worth to you, but understand you may not be able to do what everyone else can do. What's appropriate for a young dancer of 17 is not the same as for a woman of 35.

questions, without options. It's the rare ballet teacher who will ask the class if they prefer doing *piqués* or *passés* that day! If you don't feel like doing *adagio* today—too bad. If you can't handle following orders, don't take the class.

Are we exaggerating? Perhaps a little to make a point—but it's a sound one. With a discipline like ballet, which traditionally begins in childhood, you have to expect some infantilization in the way that a traditional class is organized and taught. For the adult, it means tuning into a different mind-set, a different set of expectations.

At the same time, as an adult, gratifyingly, you do have choices. And one of the keys to pleasure (and progress) in an adult ballet class is to find a teacher who adapts traditional teaching so he or she doesn't treat you like a recalcitrant six-year-old. Your ballet teacher should respect you as an adult and understand that you are competent in other areas of your life where he or she is not. Remember, this is adult ballet. You're there because you want to be—not because your mother signed you up!—and you have the right to shop around.

LEARNING WITH MIND AND BODY

Teaching adults is very different from teaching children or training aspiring professionals, and you should find a teacher who understands and appreciates the differences. This does not mean, however, settling for a watered-down version of a ballet class. Many students at the Joffrey Ballet School said they'd felt patronized by more exercise-oriented classes, masquerading as ballet; they came to the Joffrey program because they wanted real technique, real ballet, according to faculty member Dorothy Lister, a long-time teacher of adult ballet. "Adults want to be taught the correct way, and they deserve that. They have the right to be exposed to the very best training, and it's up to the teacher to take the adult to his or her full potential," she says.

Lister points out that in many cases, that potential may be surprising. "I taught one boy who was 25 or 26, and the next thing I knew he was dancing at the Met and choreographing small shows and nightclub acts," she recalls with pleasure.

One of the most obvious differences between teaching children and adults is that adults understand anatomical and directional references. This means that it's seldom necessary for a teacher to use his or her hands to physically correct an adult's positioning. "Adults are not always as approachable, in terms of physical corrections, as children may be," points out Kulyk, whose distinctive style often has him crawling around on the floor assiduously correcting feet. Elizabeth D'Anna, another faculty member who, as a teenager, studied at the Joffrey Ballet School before she began to teach, may stroke a student's back and shoulders to get her to relax or have her take deep breaths. "Children have no fear. They just do it," she explains. "Adults are tighter and more self-conscious, which is why ballet is such a good release."

Individual corrections are often given during an exercise. Here, as the class begins to do grand plié, *the accompanying* port de bras *needs extra attention.*

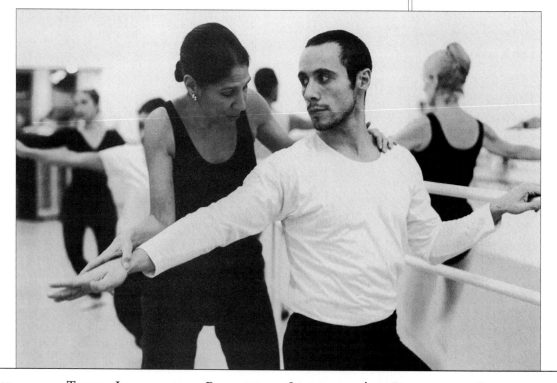

THE JOFFREY BALLET SCHOOL'S BALLET-FIT

D'Anna tries to make ballet more approachable by pointing out that many people actually do ballet movements in the course of daily life. "There are so many perfectly natural movements that pertain to dance," she points out. "When you stand on your toes to reach for something on a high shelf, it's a form of *relevé*. When you bend down to pick something up off the floor and kick your leg back, it's *arabesque*. As for swimming, that's *port de bras!*"

For adults, ballet can also be an intellectual activity. They can absorb corrections with their minds, sometimes before their muscles catch on. Abby, a magazine editor in her forties and a Joffrey adult beginner, told us that while she understands the steps in her head, when she looks in the mirror, she discovers that she's doing them wrong. "Sometimes I'm just shocked," she admits. However, one of the earliest signs of progress is the ability to self-correct in that manner. In fact, one of the first things a teacher should teach adults is what to look for in the mirror and how to correct what they see.

Unlike children, many adult beginners need an understanding of the thinking behind the movements rather than blindly adhering to rote. "Ballet is not just a physical thing, it's a mental thing with adults," says Bustillo. "The mind is the first thing to function, even when the body is not as flexible or pliable." On occasion, though, we want to stress that too much thought can get in the way of the process. Sometimes, you have to stop thinking and just let your feet do it!

For instance, adults have a history of worldly experience and are able to respond to historical or literary allusions that explain the origin of a movement or step or that illuminate a particular passage of music. "I enjoy the intellectual aspects of ballet and dance—the history, comparing styles, exploring connections," one Pennsylvania student commented. Many adults also say that their ballet classes have reawakened their love and appreciation for music, classical and otherwise. An adult beginner in Maryland says she's learned more about music from dancing than she did in all her many years of piano lessons. "My strictly recreational playing has even improved immensely, and I understand far more about different forms of music," she adds.

Frequently, in addition to an adult's cultural experience, the adult's response to class may be colored by memories of childhood ballet classes, often positive, but sometimes not. One Joffrey Ballet School student recalled a particularly brutal childhood dance teacher, "I wish I had changed teachers instead of [dreading going to class] and giving up on myself, but I was a pretty fragile child." Another student, now a dedicated Joffrey adult beginner, points out, "Adult ballet is so different from what I studied as a child." She adds, "It was such a relief to hear people laugh and joke in class, to hear steps explained with a more sophisticated vocabulary [along with] an adult description of what was happening—or maybe not happening—physically."

ASKING QUESTIONS IN CLASS

Although part of the tradition of ballet is that the teacher is an absolute figure in the class, we believe that the sensible teacher of adult ballet should allow some leeway in terms of taking questions. After all, most adult beginners are not going to respond instinctively from the results of early daily training, but rather through their intellectual understanding.

At the Joffrey Ballet School's adult classes, students are encouraged to ask questions . . . within reason, that is. Teachers often find it helpful to open the class to questions, especially when they can resolve problems that apply to most students in the room.

But lengthy personal discussions, arguments, and laments over your inability to execute a *pas de bourrée*—no way. Save it for after class if your teacher has the time, or see about signing up for a remedial private lesson.

ASSESSING THE TEACHER'S METHOD

In the final analysis, look at your prospective class with a discriminating eye. It's not a matter of distinguishing between good and not-so-good, between quality and not, but in identifying what's going to work for you personally and what isn't. Below, some pointers:

◆ Check out the teacher. Does he or she sound authoritative or authoritarian (there's a fine line here). While we freely admit ballet class is a dictatorship, do you really want to take a class from a dictator?

◆ Does the teacher make sense to you? Can you relate to the teacher's language; i.e., the metaphors and images he or she uses to explain different steps. The action of a *pirouette,* for example, is often likened to that of a spring. Pulling up—the spine-lengthening posture all dancers and dance students affect—is frequently compared to the steady tug of an imaginary string coming out of your head. Some teachers use more obscure metaphors or political images. George Balanchine frequently used analogies to cookery. In the Joffrey classes, when we admonish students not to look at their feet, we often put it this way: "It's like watching a pot of water, waiting for it to boil. It doesn't happen as long as you're looking at it."

◆ When the teacher demonstrates a step or position, can you follow? Does your teacher use hand gestures or actually get up and dance? Often adult beginners need to see an actual demonstration, while more advanced students don't. And approaches vary. Sometimes an older teacher, or one recovering from an injury, may call on an advanced student or teaching assistant for demonstration purposes.

◆ How does the teacher look? Is he or she professional and well groomed? It's important to be able to relate to the teacher. Some students may prefer a young woman; others, an older man; still others, a teacher who has a performing background.

◆ Is the teacher fit?—and does it matter to you? Learning from a teacher who is overweight can be a problem for some students. Conversely, a young teacher in Spandex-sleek shape—too trim and energetic—may be overly intimidating to adult beginners. If you're finding things difficult, it could be discouraging to have a superfit teacher.

◆ Finally, look at the other adult students in the class you're considering. Will you feel comfortable with them? Are you more experienced than the best of them (in which case you'd be bored)? Or are you hopelessly behind the least proficient? Ideally, you should be able to imagine yourself squarely in the middle after a reasonable number of classes.

Don't fall into the trap of judging the adult ballet teacher by his or her students' proficiency, however, and don't be disappointed when they don't look—and dance—like ballerinas. If your only experience with ballet is in the audience watching a professional company, seeing a beginner-level class may come as quite a surprise. "We may not look that good yet, but I'll tell you, we feel just great," one adult beginner in Seattle commented. Just remember that all dancers start out as beginners. Another adult beginner, in her late thirties, also from Seattle, told us she was actually relieved when she first observed the beginner class that she was considering taking. "I was afraid they'd all be in their teens and in great shape. Some were, but most weren't. And I thought they were pretty terrible, so I knew I'd fit right in," she recalls. After about eight months, though, she revised her opinion. "You can't believe how hard we work," she boasted. "And you know, some of us look pretty good!" Note: We have strong feelings about adult levels of ballet, by the way. Strictly speaking, all adults are beginners; some are just more experienced beginners than others.

IT TAKES CONSISTENCY!

Joffrey faculty member Elizabeth D'Anna likes to tell adult students concerned about progress that it takes time, it takes repetition, and most of all, it takes consistency. If you come to class once a week, the body and the muscles don't remember from one week to the next, even though the brain may, she explains. "The more you do, the more you can do, the more repetition, the easier it is for the body to take a correction and make it hold." For example, don't work on absorbing six different corrections at once, she advises. Instead, spend a month correcting one thing, like keeping your heel forward, or keeping your hips square. If you can manage to do that for a month, consistently, it will be fixed. Then, move on to the next trouble spot.

Making Progress: What Can Adults Expect?

As long as you continue to take class regularly, you cannot *not* improve. Just keep in mind that in ballet, progress is always gradual; it's the nature of the art. If progress is your goal, patience has to be part of your makeup. In the dance world, conventional wisdom says it takes eight years to make a dancer!

What kind of progress can the adult ballet beginner hope for? As you might expect, it's completely individual: Some students catch on more quickly than others. Yolanda, in her thirties, moved ahead at an unusually rapid pace. She became totally hooked! The only time she missed her three-times-a-week classes was for her honeymoon. After just eight months, she was clearly ready for a faster class.

On the other hand, Yuki, a beautiful adult beginner in her twenties, with a lovely and supple body, had trouble with a slightly "brittle" (i.e., not deep or elastic enough) *demi-plié.* This brittleness was affecting her *pirouettes.* It took months of patient work before she was able to execute one with ease. (It was beautiful, and she was thrilled!)

Even if you have no interest in being "promoted"—you probably want to see progress. Most adults do. One of the best things about ballet class is that no matter how inexperienced you are when you start, or what shape you're in, you can only get better.

Adults often see progress quickly in the beginning—after all, there's a lot to learn! Later, things slow down (there's still a lot to learn, it's just that the improvement is not as obvious). Keep in mind that ballet class is not like going to the gym and lifting weights, where you may advance from five-pound barbells to ten, then to twelve-pounders. It's not goal oriented, it's process oriented, and you've got to enjoy the process. Still, however subtle it may be, progress is there whether you see it or not.

As students' strength and stamina increase and they begin to accomplish basic barre exercises with more ease, less tangible forms of progress come into play. Because ballet is an art, we discern progress in an aesthetic sense as well as in more measurable gains in strength and stamina. This means that your arms may look prettier and shapelier . . . your torso more pulled up . . . your foot pointed more naturally. Plus, you won't make as many technical mistakes. You'll still need corrections; they'll just be different ones, and you'll often be able to make them yourself.

As this happens, students often become motivated and excited, inspired to try a *pirouette* if they haven't before, or attempt a diagonal combination. Also, sometimes after many months, something just clicks—and the adult beginner may begin to achieve far more than he or she ever originally intended or thought (we've seen it happen). "To see the joy on an adult's face is just as important as seeing it on a child," one teacher commented. "It just shines right

At every level, from beginner to advanced, the ballet student (here, in attitude) improves as each new correction is internalized.

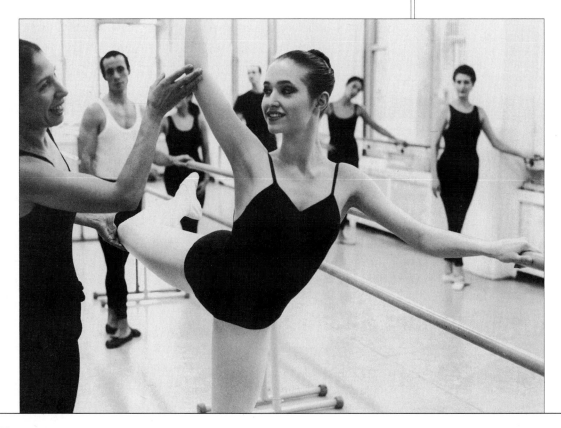

through." In fact, some adults, to their satisfaction and delight, become highly competent and find a whole new range of career opportunities, short of performing, opening up for them.

One particular Joffrey adult student in her late twenties started out with very little muscle tone. Soft and somewhat thick and flabby around the middle, she completely changed her body in just five determined months, attending class religiously three times a week. Each week, she looked visibly tighter, firmer, and leaner—even her legs looked longer (no, they didn't grow, but they looked longer)! Another Joffrey beginner, in her forties, swore that after attending class for a year, she grew a full quarter of an inch. Alas, not possible, but her posture did change—dramatically—which is where that extra quarter inch probably came from.

These changes are fairly typical of what adults can expect, depending, of course, on their starting point, how often they attend class, and how motivated they are. Bodies often appear to lengthen, and they do, in fact, tighten. Unless you're careful about what you eat, you may not lose weight, but you may look like you have, as your muscles become more toned. Keep in mind, too, that muscles are heavier than fat, so even if your weight hasn't changed on the scale, you may be losing body fat anyway.

Another change has to do with body awareness and control. There's a pride in the commitment of ballet, be it the commitment you make to show up in a leotard two or three times a week, or in the control you may gain over the way you look. In ballet class, you learn to control the way you move; you teach your body to respond—without tension, without pressure, without negativity. For one advanced adult beginner who had suffered through a terrible series of miscarriages ("My body betrayed me," she says), ballet became therapeutic, a way for her to regain her sense of physical control. "In ballet class, my body does what I tell it to," she told us.

Of course, not all adults care about progressing to the next ballet level. Some are content to stay where they are. Often highly accomplished in their professional lives, they find it a relief to be

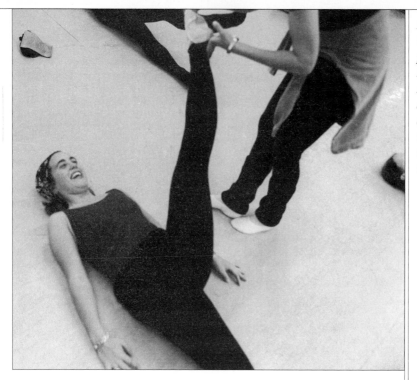

Physical changes are certainly a major part of the progress that many adults see. Many times, after only six months of classes, adults who haven't exercised in years notice that they have firmer, flatter tummies and trimmer thighs.

able to learn for sheer pleasure without the pressure to excel.

For example, although she could easily take a faster class, Kathleen, an accomplished adult beginner, prefers staying with a particular teacher, who conducts a slower, more deliberate class at a pace that allows her to perfect her movements. Francine, another student, put it this way: "I have so much competition in my working life that I enjoy having at least one area of my life where competition and progress are not the point."

So if you find a class that appeals to you and that you find relaxing and enjoy attending—even its time schedule is reasonably convenient!—stay with it as long as you are comfortable working at a slower level than you are capable of.

THE TYPICAL BALLET CLASS

1. At the barre (warm-up stretches, optional): classic barre exercises beginning with *pliés*, to tone muscles, build strength, increase flexibility, and improve coordination

2. On the floor (optional): strength-and-endurance-building exercises to isolate abdominal and leg muscles

3. In the center: *adagio*, turns, jumps, and combinations to teach balance and coordination (and also provide some cardiac benefits).

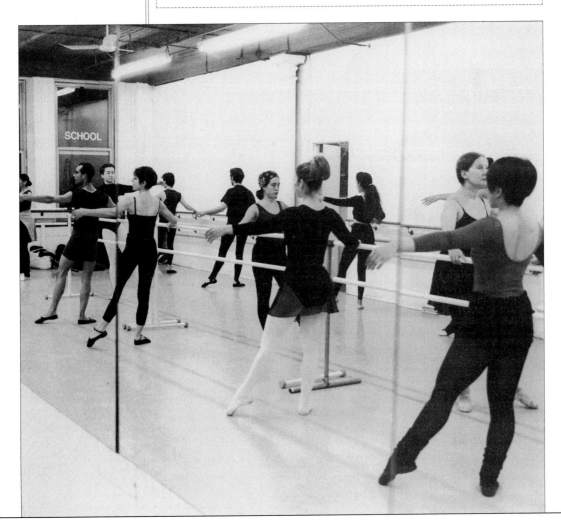

Starting Out: What to expect . . . and why

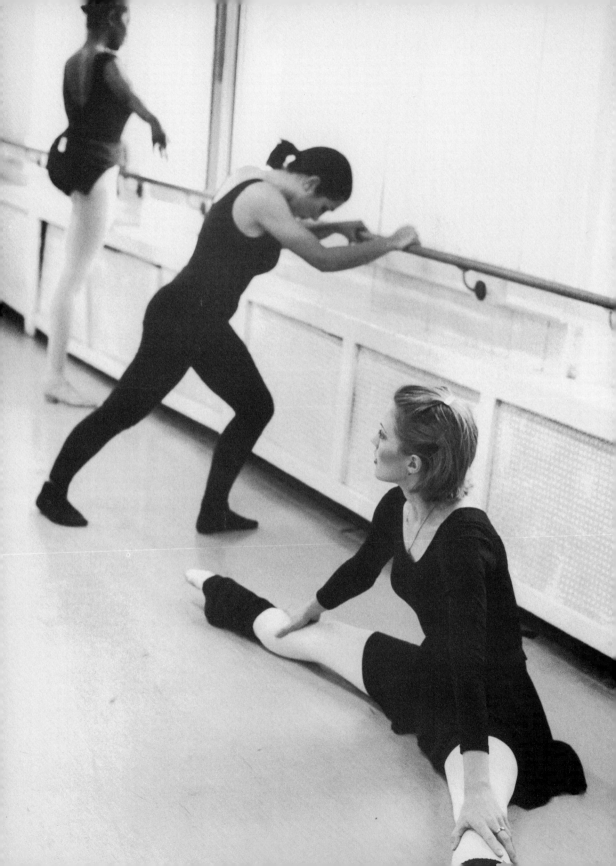

3

$\mathcal{G}$etting Physical

$\mathcal{e}\!\!\!\sim\!\!\!\cup$

THE BALLET BODY

THERE'S NO QUESTION that the professional dancer's body is an enviable thing. Long and supple, slim yet strong (and almost appallingly flexible), it's a body that moves, that can do things, that has vitality and energy and control. And it's thin . . . we have a lot to say about how thin, bearing in mind that dancers' bodies—in the skimpiest of bodysuits and tights are subject to intense scrutiny, on stage and off.

We tend to idealize the dancer's body. How it appears to move effortlessly in ways that are inconceivable to outsiders. Their legs shoot up to nearly 180 degrees. Their leaps defy the laws of gravity; they hover in the air, as if suspended by invisible strings. Small wonder that in the early days of the art, ballerinas were considered exalted, almost other-worldly creatures: weightless, boneless, enveloped in ethereal gauze and illusion.

ARE YOU BUILT FOR BALLET?

Different body types excel at different sports and pastimes. With each body type there are hallmarks of particular types of exercise. You can tell when a woman is into lifting weights or a

You may have seen some professional dancers whose bodies are so gaunt they're not enviable—no matter how talented they are. They're the ones you thought of, perhaps, when you shied away from taking a ballet class (they look like 12-year-olds!). That's not the look of health and fitness we are talking about; it's the look of a finely tuned instrument for a choreographer to work on, for a costume-maker to dress. That is not our goal.

man is a dedicated runner. Champion gymnasts are tiny and lean with small frames. Yoga practitioners are often very flexible, but they can't move (except, perhaps, for "power yoga," a relatively new yoga form, there's little or no natural flow of movement in the art).

Just as you can spot a swimmer a mile away (the broad back, wide shoulders, and muscled, sinewy arms), a dancer looks like . . . a dancer. So do dance students, and after a while, so will you. When you see former dancers, regardless of age or however many decades ago they studied, you can tell they've had ballet training by their carriage and by their long, lean line. This, by the way, has nothing to do with their weight. One former dancer we know who's no longer slim still has "the look." No, it's not the hair bun, but the underlying muscle tone, the way she moves and carries herself. You don't have to starve; you don't have to develop eating problems; you don't have to look sick or be stick-thin, to look like a dancer.

For professional dancers, it has been said that anatomy is destiny. Ballet on a performance level is far too demanding unless you've got the ideal build—and feet—and there's a laundry list of specific qualifications (both aesthetic and athletic), including sloped shoulders (which make the neck look longer); loose hips for a wide turnout; long, slender arms for women; and, also for women (men do not work *en pointe*), short "even" toes for *pointe* work, a flexible foot (but not too flexible—too high an arch may make *pointe* work difficult), and other qualifications.

In recent years, there's been some movement away from a uniform look in ballet companies toward more diversity of body types (as in modern dance or ethnic companies). It's a movement that, on the whole, we applaud. Still, common sense dictates that certain physical characteristics—flexible feet, a wide turnout, a slender build—will always remain professional standards.

For adult ballet students, of course, it's a different story. For example, if you've got short legs and a long torso, don't expect the long line in *arabesque* that comes with long, slender limbs. On the other hand, with shorter limbs (and, consequently, shorter muscles), you may have better balance and body control (your center of gravity is lower to the ground), as well as the ability to turn and jump more easily and with more power. Just be sure to stretch, not only to maintain your flexibility, but to keep short muscles from becoming bulky.

Other factors: A small frame (with small, light bones) may aid in the quickness that larger, bigger-boned dancers lack; if you've got a tight Achilles tendon (one of the most vulnerable parts of the dancer's body), deep *demi-pliés* will be harder, if not impossible, to achieve without lifting your heels, which in turn, can adversely affect your jumps. Strengthening the calf and foot muscles, stretching the whole lower part of the leg, and learning to use it all together properly can help compensate for this.

A "looser" body—that is, one with hypermobile joints and flexible muscles—will often take to ballet more easily. This body type tends to need less warm-up than someone who is naturally stiffer (the flip side of being loose is that you usually need more work on control and strength, and you may also be injury prone).

Conversely, someone who is less flexible, with less "stretch" in the muscles and less "play" in the joints, will need more time for stretching and warm-up but often has more stability, strength, and control. For example, *adagio* and jumps can be especially demanding. And don't forget strong abdominals to help hold you erect and help support the back.

Gail Grant, author of the indispensable *Technical Manual and Dictionary of Classical Ballet* (Dover Publications), and other writers on ballet frequently point out another intriguing anatomical consideration: whether a dancer's legs tend to be *arqué* (bow-legged) or *jarreté* (knock-kneed). Before you protest that you're neither one, let us point out that these are very subtle conditions. It's the rare set of legs, professional or otherwise, that are completely and symmetrically straight!

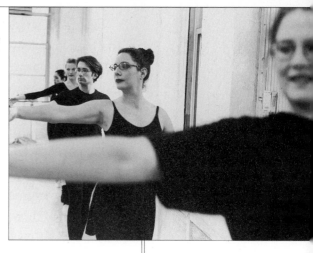

Dance students whose legs are *arqué* are generally tighter, strongly built, but stiff; while their legs don't go up that high, they're usually better jumpers. How to tell: Stand with your feet together and parallel, heels and toes facing forward. If you're *arqué*, there's a space between your knees.

Dancers whose legs are *jarreté* are the opposite. They often do a beautiful *adagio* but they don't jump as well. How to tell: When you stand in first position, your knees touch but your heels won't.

On stage, you'll see dancers who are *arqué* as well as those who are *jarreté*. Either type of dancer may also be hyperextended (i.e., their knee joints bend backward). Hyperextension is a look that's especially apparent—and admired—on stage, particularly in dancers whose long, coltish legs tend to be *jarreté*. Strictly speaking, though, hyperextension is not "correct."

BEYOND THE MIRROR: GETTING PAST THE IMPOSSIBLE IDEAL

Inevitably, for adults deciding to take up ballet, the image of the ideal dancer's body prompts insecurities about one's own—the shape you're in, the shape you want to be in, and, if you're over 40 (or 50), the age you are.

Taking up adult ballet means getting past measuring yourself against an impossible ideal (i.e., the professional dancer's body—which is most assuredly not the result of two hours a week of exercise!). It is realizing that in the end, the numbers on the scale may be less important than the ability to move with grace and confidence and the desire to make exercise and fitness through ballet a regular part of your life.

One of the factors we want to stress to adult ballet students is not to judge themselves by what they see in the classroom mirrors, which at many schools and studios may have distortions all their own. At the Joffrey Ballet School, for example, students who are in the know place themselves in front of "the thin mirror" and as far as possible from "the fat mirror" in certain classrooms.

Although dancers on all levels are self-critical, many adult dancers, particularly those in their forties and over, tend to put themselves down for not reaching a youthful ideal. This is especially prevalent among adults who have taken ballet as children or teenagers and who return at a later age. "You can't pick up where you left off," one teacher sensibly advises. "You can't go by what you looked like—or what you could do when you were younger. Expectations have to change." Most, in fact, would be wise to take a cue from one adult beginner, a 63-year-old grandmother and legal secretary who began taking class a year ago as a relief for her arthritis (and has lost nearly 30 pounds, down from 295, in the process!). She wisely reminded us that "there is something in ballet class for everyone; I have the ability to stay on my feet for much longer periods of time; I have more energy; I don't tire as easily."

RESHAPING YOUR BODY

Okay. You're convinced that you want to take ballet. You may even be eyeing a leotard and slippers in your local dance shop (see chapter 4). But how does ballet class rate as an exercise? What is it going to do for your body and how is it going to do it?

As an activity, adult ballet as the cornerstone of your fitness program is amazingly complete. Many physical activities provide you with one, maybe two benefits along with a handful of negatives. For instance, if you're building strength by lifting weights, you're not doing much to improve your flexibility or to get aerobically fit by working your heart and lungs. Nor is it the best and most effective way to burn calories. If you're into stretching only, you're not developing strength or balance or endurance. While running elevates the heart rate, it mainly works the lower body (not to mention the high risk of injury due to joint impact that comes along with it).

But with adult ballet, you have—almost—a total fitness package. Ballet is a low-impact, nonjarring activity that, unlike conventional aerobics or weight training, lengthens rather than shortens the body's muscles; increases rather than inhibits mobility; and, if you exclude jumps and *grands pliés,* even eliminates most joint stress.

Ballet builds muscles that are strong, not bulky (muscles can bulk up if you're not working correctly, so a vigilant teacher is important). It increases endurance. It's downright fabulous for flexibility, coordination, and balance—besides being an excellent way to strengthen the abdominals to improve spine support. It may even help the circulation to your working muscles as you learn to use your body properly as a smoothly functioning whole.

Of course, ballet is not perfect. While it does provide some cardiac benefits, admittedly, unless you're working at a performance level, it's not aerobic (meaning: it's not one of those non-stop activities that conditions the heart by raising its rate high enough for sustained periods of time to make a significant difference).

But it does provide just about everything else. If you're already healthy and active, use ballet to stay in shape; or, with another form of exercise, to get in shape.

In short, a good twice-a-week adult ballet class, combined with the surgeon general's latest recommendation of 30 minutes of daily aerobic activity (walking briskly, swimming, climbing stairs, cycling, jumping rope), should give you all the exercise you need.

Increase it to class three times a week, and you'll feel healthier than ever before. Stick with it and the payoff will be worth it: buttocks and legs that are strong and toned, shapelier arms, a tighter, more flexible midsection, impressive posture, plus lean, flat abdominals that are better trained for their daily tasks of stabilizing the torso and supporting the lower back.

Of course, your age and your starting physical condition (how active you've been previously) will influence, to a great extent, what you can expect and how fast you'll progress when you first start out.

It goes without saying that you can't change your basic body structure or your bone size. You can't make narrow shoulders broader, short legs longer, or broad hips narrow. But to dwell on what you can't do is to miss the point. It's nothing compared to what you can do, if you combine the strength-building, muscle-stretching, body-toning powers of ballet with an aerobic exercise (neither one works alone) and, of course, a healthy diet. You can change your body's ratio of fat to lean; you can firm and tone your muscles. Keep in mind that your age, your work load, your stress level are supporting factors—as is the amount of time and commitment you are willing to put in—but in short, ballet can reshape your shape. We've seen it happen.

RATING BALLET AS EXERCISE

Strength

◆ Ballet builds strength gradually by working most of the major muscle groups, including the quadriceps, hamstrings, gluteals, back, shoulders, and especially the abdominals.

Strength also comes into play in the floor exercises, given in many classes, and in the jumps that ballet routinely calls for. Even in executing the simplest exercises at the barre, you're constantly pulling up, working the abs. Note: It's this healthy "strength training" that helps prevent the muscle and bone loss that begins during your twenties and thirties. And when you increase your strength, you improve your muscle mass, which in turn increases your ability to burn fat and calories.

Endurance

◆ Muscular endurance is built by continuously challenging the large and small muscles of the body. While muscle strength is measured by the amount of resistance a muscle can take (for example, the force and power you can generate in a single movement, as with a jump), muscular endurance is the ability of your muscles to do it again and again and again; i.e., to jump repeatedly without tiring. You know you've reached the limits of your muscular endurance when, on the 10th repetition of an exercise, your legs feel like they weigh 400 pounds every time you lift them off the floor. But over time, and with consistent effort applied in small increments, ballet students usually find they're able to handle more, work longer, and work harder. You know you've got endurance when you can whip through 32 *changements* (jumps in fifth position in which you change feet), then continue jumping without giving out. In any case, when you finish your class feeling energized—rather than exhausted—you know you're on your way.

BALLET-FIT TIP

Adults practicing the *Ballet-Fit* floor exercises at home who want the challenge of working against even more resistance can try wearing light (three-pound) ankle weights when doing leg lifts, *entrechat sixes* (on the floor, as part of the floor exercises), and *ronds des jambes en l'air*. Before wearing them in class, however, check with your teacher. He or she may not find them appropriate.

We've been talking about muscular endurance, but there's also cardiovascular endurance (your heart and lungs are responsible for this), which means how long your body as a whole can last through a designated activity, sport, or aerobic test and how hard your heart has to work. You'll see improvement here, too. You won't huff and puff quite so much by the end of class (or after doing those 32 *changements*).

Ballet develops both kinds of endurance. In terms of muscular endurance, your own body weight is used as resistance against gravity. As for cardiovascular endurance, when you stop panting after a series of jumps, you'll know your system has adjusted, and, more likely than not, your heart and lungs can tolerate a full hour of class. Note: If you want to check out your working heart rate at a glance in ballet class, pick up a heart-rate monitor. You can get one in most athletic equipment stores.

Flexibility

◆ Flexibility has to do with your range of motion—another component of balanced fitness. The increased flexibility that ballet pro-

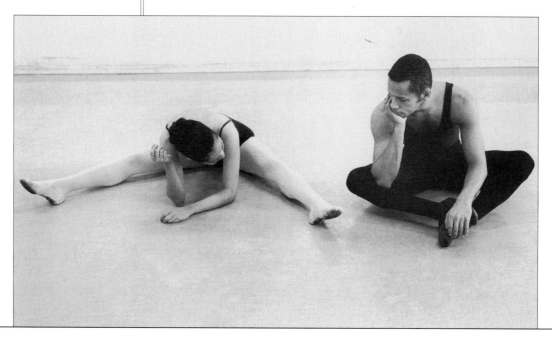

vides in the long term not only allows you to move freely but helps keep your muscles relaxed, which in turn prevents muscle tension and prevents injury.

How flexible you are is determined by the elasticity of your muscles and tendons, the length of your ligaments, and the configuration of your joints, which can vary throughout your body. One adult ballet beginner we know can hoist her legs almost as high as she could when she was captain of her high school cheerleading squad, but her back mobility is limited.

Some women may find that they're less flexible at certain times of the month, depending on the fluctuations of their hormones, or that their balance may be off due to monthly water retention. You may start to notice this after you've been taking class for a few months and begin to become more aware of your body.

Many women continue taking ballet class when they're pregnant, always with their doctors' permission. Early pregnancy might

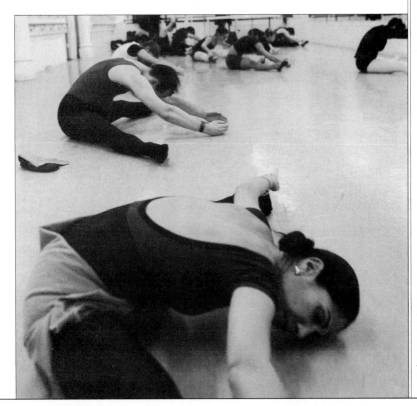

Flexibility improves with stretching exercises in class. For this stretch, it's more important to keep your back flat than to reach the floor.

be less comfortable for a variety of reasons—as may be the last few months—but the second trimester, again, with your doctor's permission, can be ideal.

Some of us are more flexible than others, but your flexibility can be noticeably improved, even if you can't touch your toes or do a split. Note: Experts tell us that the loss of flexibility some people experience as they get older may have more to do with inactivity or lack of movement than any organic factor.

The stretch you get with ballet not only feels good, it's got a long list of good-for-yous: Getting, and staying, flexible decreases the chance of muscle strains and sprains (damage to ligaments), helps maintain strength and improves posture, and protects against joint injury. Baby-boomer women take note: Increased joint flexibility—along with weight-bearing exercise—is also a preventive measure against osteoporosis, the decrease in bone density that can cause bones to become brittle, which can lead to increased bone fractures. Keep in mind that we're talking about gentle stretching for flexibility; always breathe deeply, no bouncing, no jerking, and hold each stretch slow and steady for 15 to 30 seconds. If the music is too fast, complain!

Balance

◆ Better balance is part and parcel of the improved body awareness that comes with taking ballet. You may start out looking at your feet, but after a while (six weeks, six months, it depends on you), you will learn how to place your body where it has to be to accomplish the movement without checking on yourself. That's because balance is taught, not obviously but subtly, in the weight-shifting exercises you do at the barre. "Find your balance," your teacher will demand as you raise yourself, tentatively at first, in *relevé*. "Now, take your hand off the barre." If you analyze the movements of the basic barre, it will immediately become apparent that you're constantly being challenged to figure out where your weight has to be and how to put it there. (We're talking about the standing leg here, which sounds obvious, but isn't always that easy to accomplish.)

Is balance important in real life? Unquestionably, especially as we age and may become more subject to falls. But knowing where to place yourself, how to move and shift your weight, relates directly to balance and, hopefully, to a safer old age. Which brings us to . . .

Coordination

◆ If you don't start out coordinated, ballet can help, because every ballet exercise is an exercise in coordination. Think about it: When you stretch your leg and foot in a simple *tendu* at the barre—three to the front, three to the side, three to the back, then to the side again—it's as much a matter of coordination as it is of proper weight shifting, turnout, and pointing your foot.

Just when you feel your coordination is falling into place, some teachers may complicate matters by adding arm and head movements to a combination. Some teachers may add more movements than the adult beginner can handle right away. That's why it's important to take a graded class, so that coordination of the head and arms are introduced gradually and appropriately. Classes designed for the beginner usually demand less in terms of coordination.

RECOGNIZING ADULT LIMITATIONS

After the age of thirty or so, many people begin to experience a diminishing of muscle suppleness; after forty, the fluid between the disks in the spine may begin to dehydrate, and muscles actually start to lose strength.

That's why the responsibly run adult beginner class has to emphasize safety, which means preparing carefully or avoiding certain movements altogether, for example, big jumps (like *grands jetés*) that require landing on one leg, splits, or stretches on the barre, all of which can lead to injury. Because older muscles may be less elastic, they may also be more injury prone. Less elasticity calls for keeping the muscles warm to increase pliability which means taking time for a solid warm-up at the beginning of class and cool-down at the end.

Taking class safely also means alerting your teacher to any previous injuries or present limitations you may be working with so the teacher will know how much to ask of you and whether to steer you away from certain movements or positions.

Adults, especially those who haven't exercised regularly for a while, may also tire more easily. "I find it hard to make it through the entire hour and a half class," admits one 44-year-old adult student. "I just don't have the stamina. Ballet is strenuous, even though it's stop and go, stop and go."

When students are tired, they can become careless, less aware of their bodies, and that's when injuries happen. If you've had a long day at the office and are absolutely exhausted, think twice about taking class. Learning a new combination can take mental and physical energy you just don't have. We're not saying skip it; sometimes a class can energize you. We are saying, use your good judgment.

If you are injured, stay home and take care of your injury until it heals. Dancing on an injury prolongs recovery time, makes complete recovery less certain, and can be painful and limiting. Make your comeback to ballet class two weeks later rather than earlier—in the long run, you'll be glad you did.

IF YOU HAVE BAD KNEES, A BAD BACK, AND MORE

Anyone interested should try an adult beginner class. According to Evie Vlhakis, our consulting physical therapist and an adult ballet student herself, most ballet movements can be attempted with the supervision of a qualified teacher. Katherine, an Atlanta homemaker and former long-distance runner, is a case in point. She came to ballet after being sidelined by foot surgery three years ago and now takes ballet class four times a week. "I needed a form of exercise that bestowed positive benefits without making physical problems worse," she told us.

The important thing is to listen to your body—carefully! If a joint can't bend or straighten properly, move it within your available range of motion. If a muscle (that's the center of a limb) feels tired, achy, quivery, or sore, take a break and don't worry: It's just working really hard. If a tendon (the ropy, thick end of a muscle that connects to the bone) feels like it's burning or pulling, stop trying so hard and go through a more thorough stretch/warm-up next time you take a class.

If you have bad knees, stay away from *grands pliés.* Substitute *demi-pliés,* which stop at the halfway point. Also take care with turnout: Work with what you have; don't strain. If your hips are tight, don't place your feet in an overly turned-out position; your knees may suffer. Do what is comfortable for you, making sure that your kneecaps are aligned with your toes in *plié.* If you hear a low-grade crunching or grinding sound when you *plié,* and it gets louder or starts to cause pain, stop the *plié,* rest, and wait for the

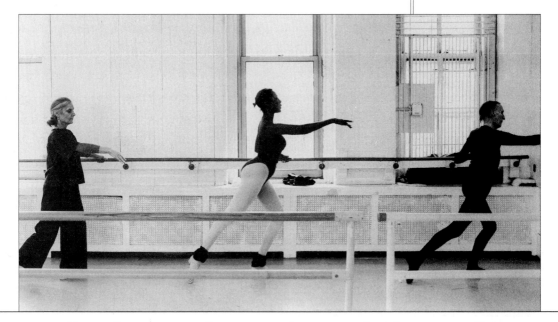

THE JOFFREY BALLET SCHOOL'S BALLET-FIT

next exercise. Note: This is a far different feeling from the more familiar popping or cracking you may hear from your knees when you're first warming up in *plié,* which is the equivalent of cracking your knuckles and is no cause for alarm.

If you have a bad back, you may experience difficulty or pain with the forward or backward bending motions, such as when your teacher asks you to *cambré* forward. Instead of thinking of *cambré* as a downward bend, think of it as a reach, and you'll be better off. If you have a joint or disk problem, or degenerated disk in the lower back, rotating your upper torso with an extended back should be avoided. Floor exercises and abdominal strengthening should be executed with special care to avoid back strain and may be difficult, since back problems are usually accompanied by weakened or insufficiently developed abdominal muscles. (See chapter 7 for ab-isolating exercise suggestions that won't strain the back.)

If you are very tight (inflexible muscles) and stiff (hypomobile joints), use ballet as an adjunct to your daily exercise program. If your ballet class isn't as "stretchy" as you would like, don't rely on it exclusively to improve your overall flexibility. Your class may focus more on the turnout muscles. In any event, it's always a good idea to stretch a bit before class. (See page 150 for stretches to add to your daily routine.)

If you are generally out of shape, weak, or in pain from other specific physical conditions but want to try ballet, talk to your doctor, physical therapist, or personal trainer about your specific circumstances (i.e., pregnancy, osteoporosis, injuries of various sorts). There's usually no need to rule out ballet class as a supplement to a regular exercise program. For women who have osteoporosis, ballet, which improves balance and offers weight-bearing benefits, can be the ideal supplement to a more extensive program of weight-bearing exercises. If you have arthritis, ballet can be your low-impact exercise (alternating with exercises designed to strengthen the musculature surrounding a problem joint). For those of you who find ballet exercises generally difficult and have a hard time with the various elements of balance, strength, and coordination, consider interweaving a yoga class with ballet in order to help develop all these areas—and to relax, too.

INJURIES TO AVOID

◆ Ballet feet: Obviously, ankle and foot problems are a common ballet ailment as one becomes more advanced. Foot problems like bunions, chronic sprains, and tendinitis can be aggravated. If your feet ache and worsen in certain positions, don't fret. A good sports podiatrist can help with inserts and taping techniques to help with your alignment.

◆ Ballet backs (i.e., disk or facet joint strains or pinched nerves) may worsen with bending forward, backward, and sideways (torso rotation), so avoid whichever positions reproduce your symptoms. And be careful with leg raises (like *battements*), which use the hip flexor muscles. These can pull on their attachments to the lumbar vertebrae. Note: you cannot safely strengthen the abdominals by performing these actions with the hip flexors; you must be conscious of the abs (we suggest putting your hands right on the ab muscles while you're doing your leg lifts so you can actually feel them working). Also, a good lumbar stabilization and abdominal program can help here, too.

HOW TO KNOW IF YOU ARE DOING TOO MUCH, TOO SOON

Listen to your body. And pace yourself. If your legs begin to tremble or feel wobbly, stop; if you feel exhausted or even dizzy before the class is over, stop and sit out the rest of the class. If you're out of shape, it's best to proceed gradually, rather than pushing it. If you're in class and something hurts, stop doing it immediately: Pain is your body's way of telling you something is wrong. Joint and muscle sprains and strains come about when you're demanding more—more strength, more flexibility—than you have to give.

This is not to say that when you first start out, if you haven't been exercising, you're not going to feel it, that mild, not unpleasant muscle soreness that tells you you've been working. You will—afterward. (When asked about physical changes she's noticed since beginning ballet about a year ago, Jennifer, a 29-year-old writer, noted: "Pain all over.")

If that's the case with you, don't start off attending class every day. It's better to give the muscles and tendons a day or so in between to recover. Feel free to stretch once or even twice during the course of the day, though; it's safe and highly recommended. Just don't stretch full out first thing in the morning. As any dancer will tell you, it's best to stretch when the muscles are most warm. If you want to start your day with a good stretch, begin slowly, gradually working up to the stretches that are more demanding. Don't start out by attempting a split! Bending forward loosely and easily is a better way to warm up.

If you begin to feel nauseated or at all light-headed, stop. Other warning signs to watch for: shortness of breath, palpitations, faintness, double vision, tachycardia (rapid heartbeat), back pain, swelling in a knee or other joint, feeling excessively hot or cold and clammy.

If you've got a cold or fever, please stay home. No one should take class when ill. It's not heroic; it's inconsiderate.

BALLET AND DIET

While professional dancers are concerned with staying thin, they are also (or should be!) concerned with staying fit. Ballet is not an invitation to develop an eating disorder. The truth is, you can't dance if you're not strong, and you can't dance if you're not healthy.

Does the pressure to stay thin in the professional ballet world affect the adult beginner? To a certain extent, perhaps. Still, while

INSIDER'S TIP

Be aware that if you are overweight, you are not going to lose a significant amount of weight by taking ballet class unless that exercise is accompanied by a change in the way you eat.

all of us participating in ballet classes are dealing with body images, realistically, how we see ourselves in the mirror depends on who we were long before we entered the studio.

As adult students become more aware of their bodies, however, they often approach their teachers for advice on how to lose weight (perhaps ballet class has inspired you to lose the last 5 pounds you never could drop, or to work on the 15 pounds you know you should have lost long ago). In fact, weight control and weight loss were frequently mentioned by adult ballet students as one of their reasons for taking up ballet. Terry, 32, an ex-dancer, now a music producer, who gained 40 pounds in six years since quitting the dance world, began taking a daily class again at the Joffrey School, where he trained as a teenager, to speed up his progress in getting back in shape. (His goal, he says, is a "godlike physique.") Jennifer sees her class as a way to lose weight without having to go to the gym. Still others view it as a way to lose weight after having a baby.

Of course, by adding two or three ballet classes to your schedule, you are going to be burning additional calories, so even if you don't change your eating habits, chances are you will lose some weight at first. Look at that weight loss as a bonus, an incentive to get you started on a healthier way of eating, perhaps, but don't expect it to continue.

We have no diet plan to recommend. If you're serious about wanting to lose weight, see a qualified professional who knows you, knows your body, and knows your health concerns.

AN EXERCISE YOU CAN DO FOR THE REST OF YOUR LIFE

Finally, we want to emphasize that once you start attending ballet class on a regular basis, unlike running or vigorous aerobics, you can continue dancing and doing your ballet workout for the rest of your life. Ballet fitness, in fact, is increasing in popularity as older exercisers have cut back on aerobics and other high-intensity activities.

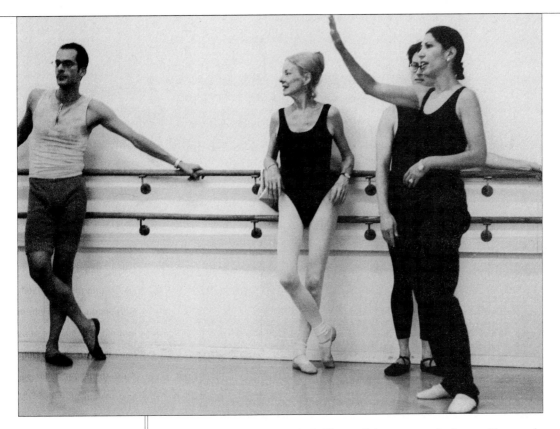

You can participate in ballet well into your sixties and beyond, as long as you allow for adequate warm-ups, rest periods, and ongoing strength-training to protect your joints. At the Joffrey Ballet School, we've taught, over the years, adult beginner and intermediate students in their sixties, seventies, and even occasionally in their eighties. We recently received a number of questionnaires from a forty- to sixty-year-old dancer's group in Maryland and were inspired by the beautiful photo of one of the adults who first began ballet twenty years ago, when she was 76!

Once you develop a reasonable degree of competence in ballet, you can continue doing the barre and floor exercises at home for your whole life. Besides, next time you're in the ballet studio, look around you: Even "old" dancers look better; they maintain their muscle tone.

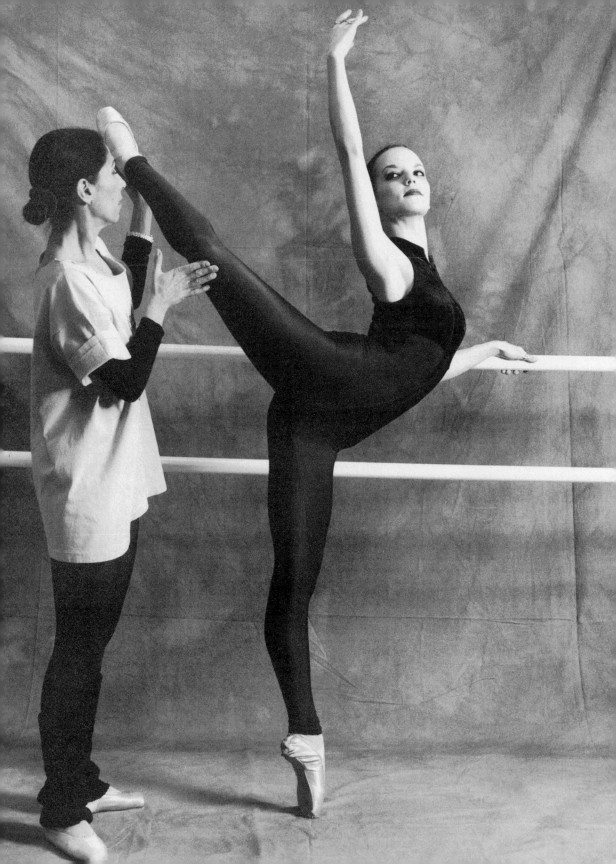

4

$\mathcal{L}$et's Get Dressed

❧

FROM YOUR OWN CLOSET

"I KNOW BALLET DANCERS wear leotards and tights. Do I have to wear them in adult classes, too?"

That's a question we hear a lot from adults who are considering coming to class—and it's a perfectly legitimate concern. The answer: The key thing for the adult beginner is comfort—and not just physical comfort, either. If you're going to be self-conscious in skintight Spandex (or whatever), you're not going to be able to relax and enjoy your class, or get the full benefit of it. Which is why we recommend that if you don't want to start out wearing a leotard and tights, then pick out what's more comfortable for you. A T-shirt and leggings, both reasonably form-fitting, will do just fine. And ballet shoes. You will need these after the first class or two.

What should you wear to ballet class? It's really fairly simple. In a nutshell, ballet clothes should work with your body, not against it.

- They should be comfortable—this is a must!
- They should be reasonably form fitting so that your teacher can correct your movements, yet loose enough so you can stretch and move with ease.
- They should help you beat the weather, hot or cold. This has to do with the fabrics you choose and the way you combine them, wrap them, and layer them. Some synthetics trap heat like storm windows, and while most dancewear has some synthetic component—otherwise they'd have no "stretch"—cotton and cotton blends do exist. These will breathe and absorb perspiration in ways that a 100 percent synthetic won't.

If you are too warm in class, looser cuts will also go a long way to help you stay cool. If you tend to get cold, go for layers, and peel down as your muscles warm up.

Ballet clothes should not only be shaped the way you're shaped, they should enhance your shape. The watchword is simple: nothing complicated, nothing overdone.

For instance, dancers and dance students like their necks to look longer. That's the reason they often cut or sculpt their garments around the neckline, and it accounts for the fact that most leotards don't get involved with a lot of collar. In ballet less is more; i.e., V-necks and scoop necks are better than crew necks, boat necks are better than cowls, and anything open (more skin means the look of a longer neck) is better than them all. Having your hair pulled up and away from your face adds to the effect even further. This should be required, even if it's just pulling it back in a ponytail or clipping it up out of the way, as you would if you engaged in any athletic event.

If you do want to go beyond a T-shirt and leggings and want to understand more about traditional dancewear—what works and what doesn't—then the following guidelines are meant to save you time, concern, and money: We don't want you spending time trying on and buying things that are not appropriate and that are not going to make you look and feel wonderful.

CHECK OUT WHAT'S WORN IN YOUR CLASS

Start by looking around the ballet studio before you decide what your "class uniform" is going to be. You may want to ask your teacher what he or she prefers students to wear, and, if you can, observe a class to see how the other adult students put themselves together. If your school also teaches professional students, look them over, too; aspiring dancers have a look—and style—all their own.

As you look around your school or studio, we can practically promise that you'll see it all: students in ballet wear that is neat and traditional (sleeveless black leotards, pink tights); makeshift (T-shirts and gym shorts over tights); too revealing ("fashion" leotards with fishnet midriff insets come to mind); unattractive in the context of the ballet studio (thong-bottomed Spandex or colors that don't appear in nature); or, in outfits that just look "wrong."

From your observations, you'll be able to piece together ideas that will work for you and your body. But again, keep it simple: Ballet fashion is not complicated and it's not to obsess over.

LEOTARDS

If you want to take class in a leotard, pick up at least two, even if you're only taking a once-a-week class. Leotards have to be washed after every wearing, and even the sturdiest will soon start to show signs of wear.

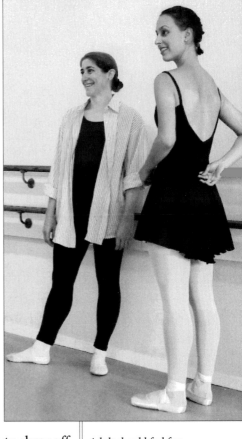

We suggest sticking with black; it's the most basic and the most popular. If you prefer a color for your second leotard, try Burgundy, deep green, blue, or a pastel (like soft, not bright, tones of pink or pale blue). In other words, the key to color in the ballet studio isn't piling on one bright color after another, it's restraint. No red, for example. For some reason—maybe because it can be distracting—it's traditional to avoid wearing red in class.

The cut and styling of leotards are the determining factors that can change the way you look and feel in them. We recommend avoiding anything contrived or "fashiony."

Sleeves (long, short, or none at all) are a strictly personal preference, but keep it simple: no puffs, nothing complicated. As a general rule of thumb, less leotard sleeve gives you more freedom of motion, but also less warmth.

As for necklines, once again, dancers like them low, to show off the line of the neck, reveal the collar bone in a fragile and feminine way. As with black-tie dressing in the "real" world, a bit of bareness goes a long way in the ballet studio.

Adult should feel free to wear whatever is most comfortable—and appropriate. Here, Kathleen and Meredith are comfortable in very different ballet-wear, but both look great for class.

WHAT CAMOUFLAGE WON'T SOLVE, LAYERING WILL

If you are uncomfortable about the way you look in a leotard, then wear a sweater, T-shirt, or workout shorts over it. Don't limit yourself to clothing specifically designed for dance or as athletic wear, either. Again, go shopping in your own closet. You can put on a man's shirt (roll up the sleeves, tie up the tail) and sweatpants, and look just fine.

We strongly suggest that female adult students wear a bra, whether needed or not. You're going to jump. Why put wear and tear on the breast tissues when it's not necessary?

In class, wear a low-backed bra and a leotard that covers it. Tip: Pin the bra to the inside of the leotard or choose a leotard that comes with a loop designed to hold the bra in place. Another option: slipping a T-shirt or cutup tights under the leotard (more on this later). It may sound strange but it works, and in the context of the ballet studio, can look very, very good.

Keep in mind that the bareness dancers and dance students like in a leotard is discreet: low-cut backs, spaghetti straps, and scooped-out necks—not cutouts in odd places. And no high-cut legs. Frequently, these ride too high on the backside, which can be an unattractive look in ballet class. A proper "ballet leg" leotard is one that's cut lower on the hip and tends to give a more natural look.

U N I T A R D S

You may not have considered unitards before, but we urge you to do so. While they were once reserved for a performance-ready body only, now they fit better than they did years ago, thanks to

SCULPTING

Sculpting is a ballet-fashion art form all its own. Because dancers often can neither find nor afford the clothing they want, they frequently end up cutting up their leotards, hacking off their sleeves, changing their shapes with a stitch or two, or just generally "sculpting" the garments to their specific needs. To enhance a small bust or lengthen the look of the neck, for instance, students may shirr a scoop-necked leotard by making three or four horizontal pleats in the neckline to create a small V. It's not a big deal, and it gives a softer, more feminine look.

fabrics that have a certain degree of hold that makes them more "forgiving." Unitards are also super comfortable and can be flattering to many different body types because they don't cut or bind at the waist or elsewhere.

Tips on Tights

While no one will dictate to an adult student what he or she has to wear, pink tights are preferred and here's why:

• Pink tights are more professional. Pink is what dancers wear on stage, and schools training professionals (like the Joffrey Ballet School) usually require their serious students to wear pink tights. Even though adult students are not professionals, they do tend to emulate them.

• Pink tights are more practical. They allow your teacher a better view of the articulation of your leg muscles so he or she can correct your positioning.

• Pink tights are more flattering. Worn with pink ballet shoes, they create a long unbroken line and the illusion of a longer leg. (Ballet shoes are pink because they emulate *pointe* shoes, which, unless they're custom-dyed for a performance, are always pink.) Please don't wear pink tights with black ballet shoes—it's an ugly look (and very unprofessional) that cuts the line of the leg and immediately labels you as a newcomer.

Even though adult beginners aren't professionals, in the ballet studio, we try to model ourselves after a professional look. Incidentally, we've noticed that as adults improve as dancers and become more comfortable in the ballet studio, they tend to come around and see the inherent wisdom—and tradition—of pink.

Still, we are talking about adult classes—you can really wear whatever you want. For adult beginners at least (never for serious students), black tights have become more acceptable. We recommend black footless tights, which give you a longer line and more professional appearance with pink ballet shoes.

INSIDER'S TIP

We're big fans of what are known as "full-fashioned" tights, which have seams running down the back and have legs that are shaped like legs. As a result, they fit better and they don't wrinkle around your ankles or the vamp of your ballet shoes.

Never throw out old pink tights. If you cut off the feet and cut out the crotch, you can slip what's left over your head and wear it under a leotard for extra warmth or for some coverage if your leotard is a little too revealing. Some dance students like to wear these instead of a bra under a leotard or to line a too-sheer white leotard. They've got a lot of uses.

As for the pink cutoff feet, they're nice as socks under black footless tights. You can salvage the feet from all your ripped-to-shreds tights for this purpose.

Flesh-colored tights? No, they're for jazz dancers. Sheer pantyhose? As with black tights and pink shoes (or vice versa, pink tights and black shoes)—very, very unprofessional. Oh, one more thing: Be sure to buy tights that are especially designed for ballet class. In other words, don't wear pink pantyhose—even opaque hose are too sheer.

Finally, with all due respect to the ballet powers-that-be, we want to emphasize that in the end, you should wear what is comfortable; if you're not comfortable, you won't enjoy your class, and if you don't enjoy your class, you'll stop coming.

In time, you will evolve your own ballet look, but what really counts are the benefits your body derives from the workout, not what you wear.

Sock Logic

Accept the fact that you're going to sweat in class. To avoid possible fungus infections when wearing footless tights, we recommend thin cotton socks (white is most common, pink is nice when you can find it).

It may be hard to believe that there are guidelines needed for something as mundane as socks, but there are. We do mean thin socks. If your ballet shoes fit properly, you won't have room for a thick sock. Ankle high socklets are most flattering because there's less fabric. If you prefer knee-highs, tuck these under your tights, not over.

Note: Many dancers and dance students like to wear ballet shoes without socks on the premise that they can "feel the floor" better that way. This is perfectly valid; however, without tights or socks, ballet shoes can cause blisters, an occupational hazard for dancers and dance students.

Leg Warmers

You'll see leg warmers around the ballet studio and yes, they do look good. But if your *tendus* don't reveal you as an absolute newcomer, wearing too much ballet gear or inappropriate ballet gear for a beginner—like leg warmers—will.

The fact is, the pros wear leg warmers to keep their muscles warm, not to get them warm. They might slip them on in between acts, during a performance; they might wear them before a class starts. But in the advanced classes at the Joffrey Ballet School, they take them off once the class begins.

However, we sometimes suggest leg warmers for adult beginners, who, unless they exercise very regularly, can be stiff when they start. For the adult beginner who is new to exercise, and new to ballet in particular, leg warmers can be a way to minimize the inevitable creaking of the knees and ankles by helping to keep (not get) your muscles warm.

Warmers come in all lengths, from those that are little more than ankle warmers to others that climb right up to the thigh. If, in the past, you have suffered an ankle injury, you may want to keep just your ankles warm, in which case, look for ankle warmers. Tip: Try children's leg warmers. They work just as well and are usually cheaper!

Super-long leg warmers that go high on the thigh may look great in the ski lodge, but unless there's a specific reason for you to wear them (to cover and warm the knee for instance), they're not as effective as shorter ones. If you still prefer long leg warmers, you can fold them to get a double layer over your calves. You've doubled the bulk, but that shouldn't matter since you'll be taking them off before class starts, we hope.

If you need something more than a standard length leg warmer to keep your hip socket warm, try full-length knitted tights over your nylon ones. All types of knits work (synthetics wash well; wool is warm but may be itchy). Either way, the flatter the knit, the better, so your teacher can see your legs.

As for color, the rule of thumb is no contrast: Match your legs, which means pink or black. Hand-knitted leg warmers, sometimes striped, can be fun, but only before or after class. One very talented

DANCE BAGS

You can tell a dancer not only by her bun but by the oversized bag she carries with her. Perhaps you've wondered what in the world was in such a big bag, and will you end up carrying a big bag, too?

When you first begin your class, you may need nothing more than a small tote or shopping bag. As you become more committed to taking class, you'll find that you absolutely can't do without a change of underwear, a spare leotard, extra tights, a pair of socks or leg warmers, a T-shirt or sweater if it's cold, a second pair of shoes that you're breaking in, a water bottle, tissues, a towel and facecloth, a makeup bag in case you're going out after class (or back to the office), a hairbrush, a hair net if you need it for your bun, soap and other toiletries if you want to shower afterward. Now you know why dancer's bags are so large.

(continued on page 69)

There are some wonderful dance bags that are made of nylon and have lots of pockets (useful for separating out a damp leotard or wet towel). Some even have holders for water bottles. These bags are usually lightweight and washable and can be found in all colors (not just black and pink) at dance supply houses. Of course any tote, satchel, gym bag, backpack, or your own designer favorite will do, too.

ballet student actually walked out of class because the teacher objected to his unraveling bright yellow leg warmers, so it may be wise to keep your fashion sense discreet.

Note: The objection many ballet teachers have to warm-up garments is that some students tend to regard them as a replacement for warming up. Even with all sorts of wraps and warmers, you still have to warm up; the garments don't do it for you. If you tend to be stiff, try your best to get to class a few minutes early to give yourself some additional warm-up time.

Sweatpants, Sweatshirts, and Other Layers

Speak to your teacher about wearing sweatpants. Some teachers actually wear them themselves, and just as many make you take them off. If, for example, you've split your leotard and tights and don't have a spare pair with you, then by all means, go for it.

Sweatpants are a matter of an individual teacher's preference. If they are okay in your teacher's class, then feel free to wear them. Just be aware that you won't get the full benefit of your teacher's corrections, since he or she won't really be able to see if your knees are bent or other crucial details.

On the other hand, sweatpants have the advantage of hiding a multitude of sins—and keeping you very warm. Nylon sweatpants were popular for a while, and you may still see them in class from time to time, but again, our teachers point out that when you wear them, they can't see if your legs are straight or bent. They may also restrict your *pliés.*

The same goes for wearing sweatshirts or the rubberized work-out pants that dance students sometimes show up in when they want to drop a few pounds (that's not the way to do it!), for T-shirts, and even for the little, layered, surplice-style dance sweaters (these are for coverage if you're shy or to help keep you warm if you're cold-blooded). If you want to or need to, fine. The fact is, at

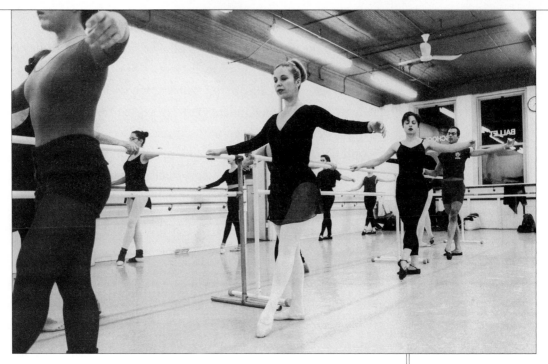

the start of class, many dancers and dance students are quite creative with their wraps and layers—around their waists, over their hips, on the shoulders—peeling down as their muscles and bodies warm. By the middle of class, the baggy sweatshirt you started out wearing may very well end up wrapped around your waist or draped across the barre.

Layers, wraps, skirts, warm-ups, T-shirts— there are lots of options for ballet class that don't require an entirely new wardrobe.

BALLET SKIRTS

Skirts don't keep you warm; they don't really hide anything, and if they do, the fabric is way too heavy. The correct length—short, just covering your bottom—is useless for anything but role-playing; we're talking about ballet's fantasy aspect here. The wrong length— that is, hovering around your knees—covers far too much. Plus, as with sweatpants, they can disguise bad habits (such as not keeping your hips square), which you're much better off correcting.

Many teachers do wear ballet skirts in class, which is why, perhaps, students adopt them, too. But teachers are often required to

Some skirt-shopping caveats: Stay away from long, bias-cut dance skirts. Some are intended for modern dancers; others for ballroom dancing; still others are just unattractive and unflattering. As in all areas of clothing, ballet-skirt styles go in and out of fashion. For example, the Russian-style ballet skirt—which wraps asymmetrically, longer in the back and shorter in the front—was popular for years; now it looks dated in the ballet studio.

wear ballet skirts: It's ballet tradition. A skirt supposedly adds to a teacher's authority (specifically with children's classes). And, yes, we admit that some do camouflage figure flaws, which is another reason some adult beginners are attracted to them.

If you insist on wearing a skirt and your teacher doesn't object, there are lots of skirts available in sheer, washable chiffon, in black or in pretty, muted prints. Keep it short, keep it matching your leotard, and maybe, in time, you'll feel comfortable enough to leave it off.

FOR THE BOYS

Men in ballet class generally wear black tights, white socks, and T-shirts. We've also seen gray tights and they look fairly nice; as for white tights, these are worn (with tunics) for performances only. In the ballet classroom, they tend to be, well . . . indiscreet is perhaps the best way to put it. If you're uncomfortable about wearing tights or don't want to invest in them right off, wear simple, narrow-legged sweatpants with an appropriate support garment (we're talking about a jockstrap).

Under tights however, a jockstrap won't do; you'll need a dance belt, which you can pick up at a good dance supply shop or by mail (see the *Ballet-Fit* Source Directory). Dance belts look like a thong and are made of black, beige, or white supportive elasticized material; the color you choose depends on the color of your tights. Is a dance belt a must? Well, it should be, even under sweats. As with any other sport, you need to have the proper equipment. A jockstrap just isn't appropriate under tights because you want to keep a smooth, unbroken line.

What else? White, black, or gray socks. Black or white ballet shoes—important, guys, you'll work better with them. One of our Joffrey Ballet School adult beginners who works on Wall Street hasn't bought his yet, but we understand. He's six foot seven inches tall and will probably need to have a pair custom-made. If you wear a nonstandard size and can't find ready-made shoes, chances are your teacher will allow you to take class in socks. By the way, ballet class is seldom politically correct—in class, you're all boys and girls. That's tradition, too.

UNDER WARES

Sports bras for women? Sure, if you need extra support and your leotard covers it. Don't wear the sports bra alone, or bra-topped active wear, without a T-shirt over it.

The wrong bra can affect your comfort in ballet class, not only in terms of the way you look but in the way you jump and move. Look for cotton or cotton blends, which are cool and absorbent (maybe with some stretch lace to help hold it in place); wide, well-placed straps that won't slip or slide; and a style that's cut low in the front, on the sides, and in the back, if you're wearing a body-baring leotard.

A bra that's smooth and without seams will also offer the smoothest line under your thinnest leotard (a front clasp will give you all-around, no bump-in-the-back smoothness). With a practically backless leotard, a backless wisp of a bra that wraps around the waist is a good idea.

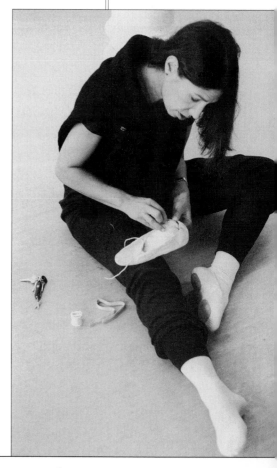

If you're busty, take class with a good supportive bra that fits; you'll feel, and look, better for it. Then lead the eye away from your bust with diversions like vertical necklines, two-toned leotards, and the like.

IF THE SHOE FITS...

While the clothes you wear to ballet class are negotiable, shoes are not. You may take your first ballet class or two in socks, but after that, you must have ballet shoes. Going barefoot is fine at

If you decide on leather ballet shoes, buy them tight. Really. Then use shoe stretch (a spray carried in most shoe repair stores) and spray them. Walk around the house on *demi-pointe* until the shoes dry and they mold to your feet. You can also cut the shoes' canvas lining out to get a better fit. The lining holds the shape of the shoe, which is not what you want. You want it to hold the shape of your foot.

home if you've got a slick floor (like linoleum in the kitchen or polished wood elsewhere), but generally bare feet run into too much friction against the floor.

Ballet shoes come in a range of sizes and styles, are reasonably priced ($12 to $30 usually), and in most brands are interchangeable in terms of "right" and "left" shoes (they're called straight lasts). They are also the only real "equipment" you'll need for class, which is quite a minimal investment, especially when you compare it to activities like skiing, skating, or tennis, where you have to acquire skis, rackets, skates, and the like. Ballet shoes are simple. They can be leather; they can be canvas; women's shoes should be pink; and they must fit properly.

Dancers spend their whole professional lives searching for the perfect soft shoe. Here's what they like:

◆ Color: Black ballet shoes are for beginners. Yes, we know you're a beginner, but don't wear them, anyway. Black shoes look terrible with the pink tights you're going to be buying (while pink shoes look perfectly correct with either pink tights or black footless ones). Guys—black or white shoes are fine and look very convincing.

◆ Size: Be prepared to try on several different brands of shoe before you find the one that's right for you; ballet shoe sizing is a world of its own. While some brands may match your street shoe size, more often ballet shoes run a good size (or two or three!) smaller than what you'd normally buy. They also have to fit snugly, more snugly than many new students imagine, which is why adult beginners show up in class with shoes that are way too big.

◆ Fit: Scrutinize the fit carefully (serious ballet students are fanatic about their shoes and you should be, too). Don't always go by what the dance store salesperson is telling you, either; not all of them are knowledgeable, we've discovered. Your shoes should be tight (they will stretch; leather a lot, canvas, less so), but not so tight that your toes curl under. They shouldn't gap at the sides or crumple at the toe.

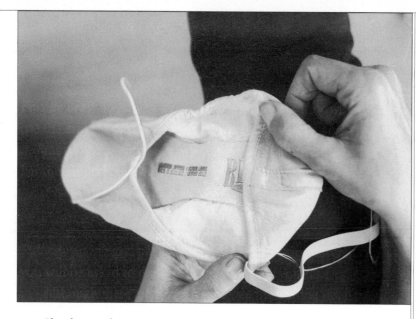

Avoid shoes that have the elastic sewn on for you. In our experience, all too often it's in the wrong place. Although it may seem logical, the elastic should not be sewn from center seam to center seam, but much farther back on the foot. How-to: Measure the piece of elastic so it fits your foot; fold the heel of the slipper forward (see photo, left); then sew in place at each corner.

Check out the vamp of the shoe; it can make a difference not only in the way the shoe looks but how you work in it. A higher vamp is good if you have very long toes; it covers them and elongates the look of the foot. If your foot is small, a high-vamp shoe may be too much shoe for your foot to handle. A low-cut vamp is usually flattering and graceful—it helps create the illusion of a longer leg—but it shouldn't be so low that it doesn't cover your toes when you're *on demi-pointe.*

◆ Sole issues: Ballet shoes are also available with split soles or whole soles. The split sole is a recent development that dancers and dance students like because it makes the shoe more flexible and gives the appearance of greater arch.

◆ Canvas shoes versus leather: Both are classic; both are correct. Leather stretches so much once you start to wear it that the fit is never as precise as we like. Canvas has the advantage of retaining its fit, it's cheaper, and you can "feel" the floor in them, but they won't last as long.

◆ Durability: How long shoes last depends on how often you attend class. A teacher's shoes, which incur extensive daily wear, may last a month before they start to get holes and shred at the

To make their favorite shoes last longer, dancers often resort to taping tricks because it's such a nuisance to break in new pairs, and the costs adds up. Between the cost factor and the comfort factor, taping is the answer!

You can repair ballet shoes by turning them inside out and using white adhesive tape over the torn spots (no one will ever know the shoes are taped). Note: Most adult beginners tend to get rid of ballet shoes well before they wear out, mostly because they don't have that much experience in buying ballet shoes and may go through several styles and brands before they find what's best for their feet.

pleating. A dancer's *pointe* shoes usually make it through a single performance only. If you're taking class one or two times a week, your shoes will probably last a year. The more you "work into the floor" (a good thing!), the quicker they'll wear out.

◆ Elastics: Ballet shoes come with two pieces of elastic, which you sew on after purchase. Before you do, bring your new shoes into class and try them on for your teacher. That way, if they're incorrectly sized (and they often are), or if they're too stiff and don't mold well to your feet (this means you'll have to work harder to point your foot), you can still bring them back.

◆ Ballet shoes are hand-lasted; this means that the charming little pleats in the front of the shoe are made by hand, and that you will see variations and imperfections from one pair to the next (even in the same size, same brand). So, even if you find the perfect fit in Capezio or Bloch's 5½ B, the next pair you buy may not be to your liking.

◆ Some older adults, especially those who have been taking classes for a while, find that they can't comfortably wear a flat shoe anymore. This is usually because of a bruised heel bone, a bone spur, soreness in the Achilles tendon or some other anomaly. They sometimes wear a pink modern dance slipper that has a thin, tiny half-inch heel. One experienced Joffrey adult beginner, Pat, a sixtyish actress, did this when she started feeling uncomfortable in conventional ballet shoes. That's fine for Pat, who takes nine classes a week—and has for years—but not for the absolute newcomer. A new adult beginner should stay with classic ballet shoes and try to work with them, unless there's some compelling medical reason not to.

◆ The little drawstring on your new ballet slippers is quite useful. It gives when you point, retracts when you flex, so your foot always looks neat and shaped. We love it, but still we prefer it stay out of sight. So tuck in the bow, please; otherwise, your pretty ballet feet will have that "Minnie Mouse" look! Look for elastic drawstrings—a nice innovation.

◆ *Pointe* shoes? Another issue entirely. Nothing we've discussed so far applies to *pointe* shoes. If you're up for your first pair—or your first pair since you were 12—turn to chapter 8.

F R O M   T H E   N E C K   U P

You don't *have* to wear your hair in a bun in class, but there are good reasons for doing so. It's neat; it's often flattering; it keeps the dancer's head looking small and elegant; it leaves the line of the neck and shoulders clear; but, most important, it keeps the dancer's hair controlled when she's turning. Technically, dancers "spot" their heads to control dizziness. This requires a sharp turn of the head, so even a neat hair braid can blind the dancer when she turns.

And, of course, it's traditional. Buns and chignons for ballet date back to the mid-19th-century to the Romantic ballets like *Giselle* or *Les Sylphides*. Today students vary the look with French

Classic ballet buns are not de rigueur, *as long as your hair doesn't get in your way.*

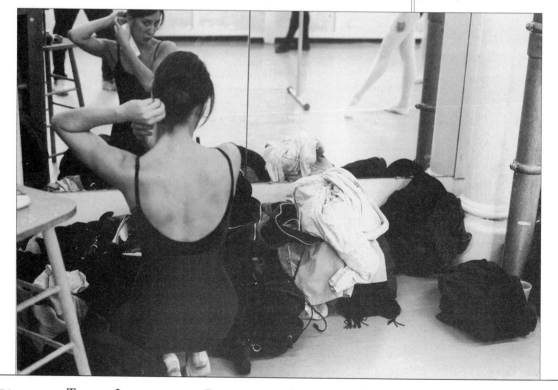

T H E   J O F F R E Y   B A L L E T   S C H O O L ' S   B A L L E T - F I T

knots, high ponytails that are braided or twisted and pinned with one big bobby pin or clip.

If your hair is long, any style that keeps it smoothed away from your face is fine. Some adult students tie their hair back in ponytails, clip it up, or wear stretchy headbands so it doesn't flop in their face when they *cambré* forward. And yes, some do wear chignons or buns.

Makeup: In class, some teachers like to see faces that are well scrubbed, while others prefer ones that are lightly made up. Since perspiration and makeup are often incompatible, if you want to wear makeup, choose waterproof cosmetics (especially mascara) or skip it entirely.

Jewelry: Leave it home. Please. If you don't wear it in class—and you shouldn't (jewelry can be dangerous, risky, distracting, and inappropriate)—it's seldom safe to leave it in your bag (unless there's a place to check valuables). If you have pierced ears, avoid long dangling earrings that could get caught in your hair and rip your earlobe; studs, tiny wires, or the smallest hoops you can find are fine. If you don't have pierced ears, avoid earrings altogether. Avoid necklaces, bracelets, and ankle bracelets. Your watch is fine, although one with a leather band may make you sweaty.

Perfume: You may have read somewhere that famous ballerinas are known by their signature perfumes, which waft across the stage in wonderful bursts of floral breezes as they turn. But in the dance studio (and especially in the dressing room), too many scents combined with the perspiration of many dancing bodies can be, to say the least, overwhelming. If you're coming to class directly from home, save your favorite scent for after class, not before.

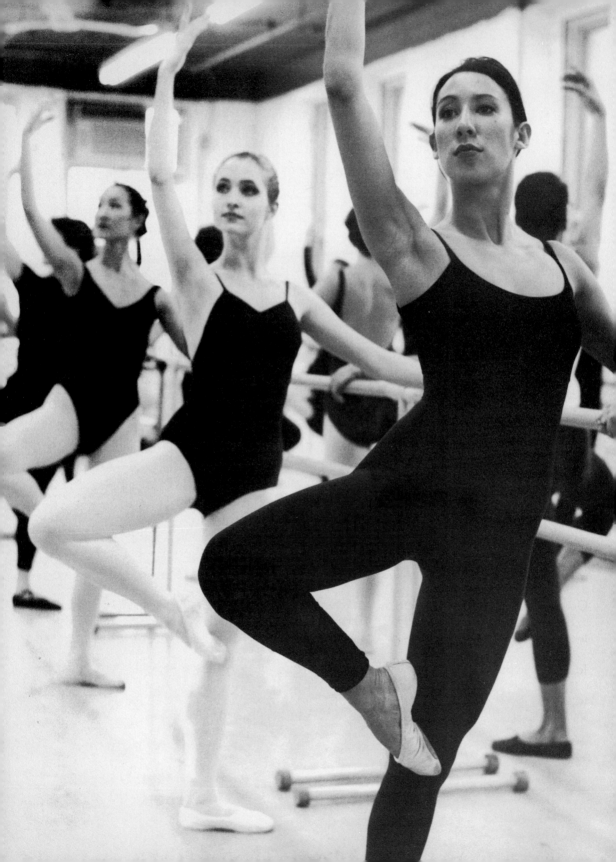

5

*T*he Language of Ballet

❧

STARTING OUT

YOU'VE CHECKED OUT THE SCHOOL, you've chosen a teacher, and, shoes in hand, you are about to show up for your very first class. What should you expect?

Of course, every school is different, but in general, you'll register at the desk where you'll be asked to fill out a form or two, sign a waiver or a routine release to protect the school from lawsuits. Then you'll be directed to the dressing room.

Change your clothes; take your bags with you; head for your class.

INSIDE THE CLASSROOM

Once you're inside the class, look around to see if there's an area where the other students have left their coats and bags. It may be on a windowsill or next to you at the barre, or, as at the Joffrey, near the piano, against the wall and away from the door. Once you've deposited your worldly goods in an unobtrusive place, find yourself a spot at the barre.

If you're new, you'll want to be close enough to the teacher to see and hear her, but not at either end of the barre. Take a spot in the middle and leave the ends of the barre for more experienced students. You will want to follow what other students do, especially when the teacher is not in view. During barre combinations, when the teacher walks around the room, watching students and making individual corrections, you won't be lost because you can follow the students in front of you or catch a glimpse of other students in the mirror.

Let the teacher know if you have special needs that may affect where you want to position yourself. Physical disabilities may require some accommodation but needn't keep you from ballet class. One Joffrey School adult was legally blind and needed to stand close to the instructor. A young student who lost an arm was still very capable in class. At the Joffrey School, there were classes for hearing-impaired youngsters, which had an assistant to "sign" the combinations and special speakers to amplify the vibrations of the music. Students who wear hearing aids are no less able to dance than those who wear glasses! We understand that there is an active choreographer and performer who takes class from a wheelchair

It's a good idea to warm up before class if you have time. Students have their favorite warm-up exercises, but should resist the temptation to stretch on the barre.

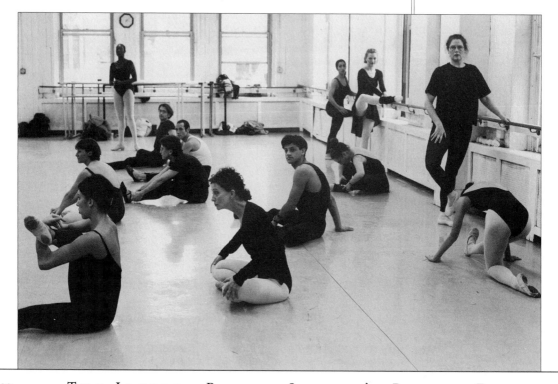

and dances with her upper body and arms. The point: Everyone is welcome.

While you're waiting for the teacher to arrive, you'll see others stretching on the floor or at the barre. Ballet students like to do all sorts of things before class to wake up the body. While class is the warm-up for the professionals, it is the performance for most students, and they want to be ready to do their best. You'll see them pointing and flexing their feet, doing *pliés* or extra abdominal work like crunches. You'll also see various contortions designed to warm up and "open" the hip sockets and increase turnout. You may be tempted to follow their lead, which is fine, but proceed with caution. No matter how tempting, don't stretch on the barre or do other extreme movements to try to open your hips. You're not warm enough or experienced enough (yet), and you might hurt yourself. For our preclass warm-up suggestions, see chapter 7.

If you've walked into an already crowded classroom with no space at the barre left, simply wait near the piano for the teacher. When the teacher arrives, he or she will recognize you as a new student and place you appropriately.

If you're inadvertently late for your first class, we suggest you just observe and take your first "real" class next time. You may be nervous to begin with, and under the best of circumstances, it can be confusing to come in after class has already begun.

FAVORITE SPOTS AT THE BARRE

Everybody tends to have a favorite spot at the barre. Some students "save" their places with a sweatshirt or towel draped over the barre; some students even tell us they get a bit disoriented if "their" spot is taken. It's not a good idea to get too attached to any one place. You should be able to take—and enjoy—class from any spot. Still, here are some pointers to keep in mind.

- Don't take a spot that someone has saved. We can't protect you from nasty looks and maybe a misplaced *grand battement.*

- Place yourself behind people who have taken the class before. How to know? Ask! Until you get to know the class, you'll want someone to follow.

- Make sure you can see yourself in the mirror so you can learn how to correct yourself and so you can see what others are doing in case you get lost.

- Don't stand at either end of the barre unless you're confident that other people can follow you. Teachers often place more experienced students in these spots; if you take one, please don't make any mistakes.

- If everyone in class is new, where you stand at the barre is less important because you're all in the same boat. *Everyone* has to follow the teacher. Note: As you become more advanced, following shouldn't be an issue anymore.

- The best position depends on you and the classroom. You'll soon develop your own preferences. But don't be surprised if the mirrors reflect a "you" you don't always recognize. The ballet studio's walls are usually completely mirrored so expect distortion. Learn which are the "fat" mirrors and try to avoid them.

- When you're doing center, being placed in the middle of the front line is a great compliment. It means that the teacher trusts you enough to let others follow you. Don't be intimidated; use center work as an opportunity to "perform." Remember, ballet is a *performing* art and classes are preparation for performing, even though that is not your ambition. If your teacher doesn't place you for center work, position yourself where you can watch yourself carefully in the mirror.

TERMS TO KNOW BEFORE YOU BEGIN

In ballet class, there are certain words and phrases you will hear over and over again. If your teacher isn't inclined to explain this basic vocabulary—and some aren't—it will be assumed that you know what he or she is talking about, or that, in time, you will absorb their meaning. To make matters more confusing, certain ballet terms may have more than one meaning; for example, *adagio* means one thing in a beginner class, another in a more advanced class or at a performance.

French became the "official" language of ballet not only because ballet originated in the French royal court but because, until the beginning of the 20th century, it was the universal language of culture: Eighteenth-century diplomats such as Thomas Jefferson and Benjamin Franklin conversed in French; in Russia, where ballet flourished, French was often the first language for the upper classes.

Literal translation of the words may help you associate the terms with the movement, but it won't tell you what to do when your teacher says *"Pas de chat,* please." Instead, translation helps you create a visual image. *Port de bras,* for example, literally means the carriage or wearing of the arms. Often the poetic relationship is subtle; you have to look closely. *Fondu* means "melted," but in the context of ballet it's a *plié* on one leg. Visually, the body appears to be "melting." The terms *pas de cheval* ("step of the horse") and *pas de chat* ("step of the cat"), and *temps de flèche* ("step of the arrow") hint at the movement, but only by poetic allusion.

Most steps are *pas* (pronounced *pah*), which means "step," or *temps* (pronounced *tahn*), which means "time." But *temps lié* (*lee-ay*), which means "tying time" (which means nothing at all) becomes more descriptive if you translate *temps* as "step." And *temps de cuisse* ("step of the thigh") stretches a literal translation by referring to the part of the leg that initiates the step.

On the following pages, you'll find some of the most frequently used terms, defined not for the pro or for the advanced ballet student, but specifically with the adult beginner—the lay reader—in mind. This is not an exhaustive presentation of the vocabulary of ballet. For that we suggest you pick up a ballet dictionary (see the listings in the *Ballet-Fit* Source Directory).

Adagio: From the Italian (after all our talk about French!). *Adagio* is an Italian musical term meaning "slow"; in ballet class, it refers to slow, stretchy exercises at the barre or in center where the student works on balance, extension, and elegance of line. For the advanced student, *adagio* also refers to partnering, also known as "pas de deux."

À la seconde: Referring to one of the five positions of the feet (see page 100), *à la seconde* means "to the side," as in "arms in second" (held open to your side), or *tendu à la seconde* (point your foot to the side).

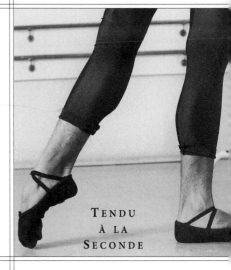

TENDU
À LA
SECONDE

Allegro: A musical term from the Italian meaning "quick." The *allegro* is the part of class (usually the second or third combination in center) when you learn small jumps. *Petit allegro* includes *assemblé,* any jump from one leg to the other; *sissone,* any jump from two legs to one; *changements,* jumps changing feet in fifth position, to name just a few of the *sautés* ("jumps") you'll learn. The large, diagonal combination at the end of class is sometimes called *grand allegro* because the jumps get *plus grand,* or bigger.

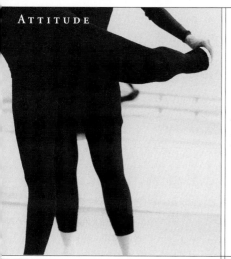

Attitude: Pronounced *ah-tee-tyood, attitude* is a ballet position in which the working leg is bent, not straight, and may be raised to the front, the side, or the back.

Barre: The barre is the wooden or metal railing that is either attached to the wall of the classroom or studio, or moved to the center, and is used as a support. You rest your hand gently on it; you don't clutch it for dear life. Sometimes, the actual exercises themselves are referred to as the barre, as in "we do the barre first."

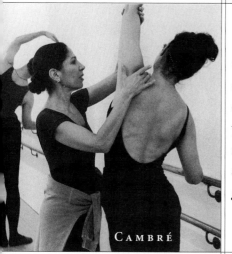

C A M B R É

Cambré: Pronounced *cahn-bray,* means "arched," but we don't really want you to arch your back when you *cambré* or bend your upper body forward, side, or back. Instead, you will learn how to pull up out of your hip sockets and reach. It's not the way you bend over when you pick up something from the floor. A circular *cambré* is called a *grand port de bras.*

Combination: Combination refers to a series or sequence of steps strung together; what a lay person might think of it as a routine. If your teacher asks you to do three *tendus* and a *demi-plié* in each direction, or three *changements* and a *relevé,* she's giving you a "combination."

Croisé: Pronounced *kwah-zay, croisé,* a part of *épaulement* (see page 88), literally means "crossed," but actually refers to positioning the body so that it is standing on a slight diagonal, or angled to present a three-quarters view to the "audience" (in the classroom, the audience is your mirror). *Croisé* and related body positions, such as *effacé,* come into play most often in center work, although in a very crowded class, some barre exercises like *grands battements* may be performed facing toward the barre on your *croisé* so no one gets kicked.

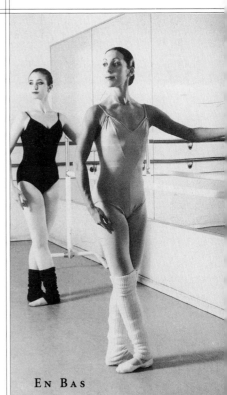

En bas: One of the positions of the arms corresponding to fifth position of the feet, *cinquième en bas* often finishes a combination. You'll be asked to do a *demi-plié* and end with your arms in fifth low, or *cinquième en bas,* as the music trails off. *En bas* arms are rounded and held low, the little fingers of each hand resting gently on your tutu, if you were in costume. Fifth high (*cinquième en haut*), the other position of the arms that corresponds to fifth position of the feet, is the same, but the arms are held up as a frame for your face. Each of the positions of the feet have corresponding arm positions; then, there are additional arm positions to complement a pose, like *arabesque.*

EN BAS

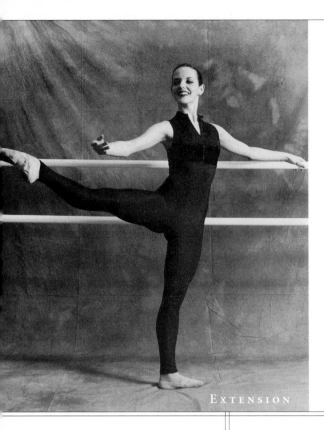
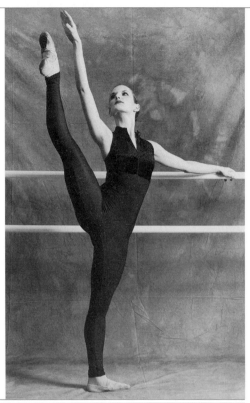

Two extensions, one lower, one higher—both are equally correct.

Extension: Extension refers to how high you can lift your leg in movements like *arabesque, battement,* and *développé.* Lifting it high may look impressive, but height is not what we're looking for in a beginner class. We're more interested in whether or not you can keep your legs straight and turned out, your hips square, your abdominals pulled.

Extension is not an indication of talent, it's a natural gift that nevertheless can be developed or improved by working on your stretch. Even without practice, most adult students can lift their legs to 90 degrees in the front (that's the angle at which you sit) and slightly less than 90 degrees to the back. But whether or not you can go past 90 degrees is not important.

En dedans/en dehors: These terms mean "inside" and "outside," respectively, and refer to directionality, because in ballet, sometimes left and right and clockwise and counterclockwise are not adequately descriptive. Dancers are expected to respond instinctively to *en dehors* and *en dedans,* but unless these words are explained, they can leave the beginner literally disoriented. We're going to simplify it: If you face the mirror, you can visualize *en dehors* as a circular movement going from front around to the back, and *en dedans,* as going from back to front.

Since so many ballet steps are circular, it's important that your teacher explains *en dehors* and *en dedans* in terms you can relate to.

En l'air: literally, in the air, or performing a movement with your leg off the floor.

Épaulement: a poetic way of describing the angles that dancers may use in facing the audience (think "shouldering" from the French word *épaules* or shoulders). *Épaulement* is said to have developed to take advantage of the shadows cast by footlights—first candles, then gaslight—which added interest and dimension to the performance.

En pointe: When a dancer is *en pointe,* she is on the extreme tips of her toes—a practice described by someone who probably never danced as "unnatural, uncomfortable, and frequently painful." The fact is, experienced dancers are completely habituated to their shoes and have their own ways of making them comfortable. No matter. It's those beribboned pink satin slippers (*pointe* shoes—sometimes called blocked shoes, but never toe shoes) that are the stuff of fantasy and dreams.

"Find Your Center": From time to time, your teacher will tell you to let go of the barre and balance, either flat or in *relevé* (on tiptoes), and "find your center." Beginners often fear that they don't have one! But it's an imaginary place somewhere around the ribcage. By locating it physically when you've "hit" a balance, you will be able to reproduce the feeling and the result, or so the theory goes.

Line: Line is very easy to see, perhaps less easy to define. It's what dancers mean when they talk about the "pattern" the body makes when it takes a ballet pose. Perhaps the best example of line is in *arabesque:* You can see the dancer's line when the leg is raised in the back and fully extended (and no matter how high the leg goes, the back remains straight). The dancer's line is broken when the leg is bent.

Marking a Combination: This means walking through a combination as practice. Before the class is required to do a combination, the teacher will demonstrate it, and students often do it with her—that's "marking" it, as if to imprint it on their muscles.

Some students prefer to watch carefully rather than mark, and some teachers don't like students to mark because they feel they're not paying full attention. But it all depends on how you learn best.

In center and across the floor, marking with another group is usually acceptable. Note: The opposite of marking is doing a step "full-out," which means full strength, not merely walking through it.

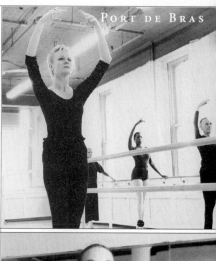

Port de bras: literally, "carriage of the arms." It's how we use the arms as part of the dance. For the beginner, *port de bras* can be as simple as moving the arms from fifth *en bas* to first and open to second position.

Pull-up: an integral part of ballet's characteristic posture; you will be asked to do it from the first class you take.

Although there are many ways to define pulling up, it might be easiest to start by explaining what it's not. It's not holding your breath or sucking in your stomach; it's not a pelvic tilt; and it's certainly not lifting up your shoulders.

One way to think about pulling up is as a readjustment of weight—lifting the weight up and out of the feet and legs and distributing it upward, articulating the abdominal muscles. Physically, what takes place is a lengthening of the area that connects the legs and the torso. This takes the weight off the feet and legs and delivers it to the torso, preferably along the spine.

Less technically, pulling up involves a feeling of "lift" or getting taller—strong and solid through the midsection, but stopping before it reaches the shoulders. Teachers have their own ways of describing pulling up. Some say flatten the abdominals; others may ask you to lift through or under your ribcage.

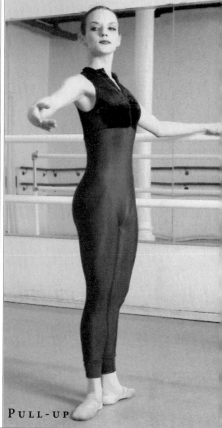

PULL-UP

Demi-pointe: not quite on the tips of your toes, but with the heels raised and all five toes on the floor.

Relevé: on tiptoes or *demi-pointe.*

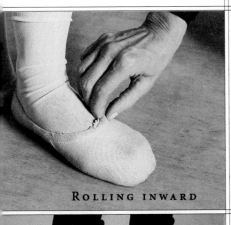

ROLLING INWARD

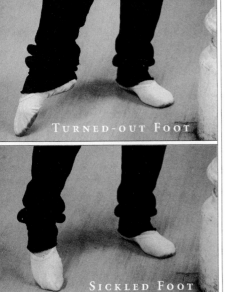

TURNED-OUT FOOT

SICKLED FOOT

Rolling inward (or outward): This very common beginner pitfall refers to the involuntary rolling of your foot toward the big toe, or out toward the little toe, depending on where you place your weight. It happens when you try to turn out from the ankle or foot, instead of from the hip socket, or when you try to work with more turnout than you have. Narrow your first position a bit if you find you're rolling in, since it places stress on the big toe joint which can lead to bunions.

Sickle: If your teacher tells you that your foot sickles naturally, don't take pride in it; it's not a compliment. But sickling the foot does come naturally to some people, often when dancers try too hard to point their feet. A sickled foot assumes an aesthetically unattractive shape in which the heel drops backward and the toes come forward to resemble a half moon or scythe.

To avoid sickling, all dancers, whether beginners or advanced, have to be constantly on the alert to keep their heels forward. We'll be giving you tips throughout this book on when to be particularly aware of sickling and how to avoid it. One way is to always think about presenting the inner part of your heel to the audience.

Sous-sus: Pronounced *soo-soo, sous-sus* is similar to fifth position in *relevé*, but the feet are held tightly together.

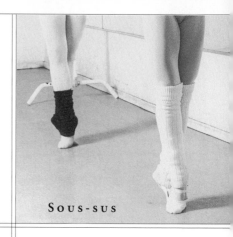

SOUS-SUS

Supporting leg/Working leg: The supporting leg is the leg you stand on (it supports your weight) when your other leg (the working leg) is pointed in *tendu*, raised in the air, or otherwise engaged. Related to this is "inside leg" (the leg closest to the barre) and "outside leg" (the other one).

TURNOUT

Turnout: Ballet is based on the concept of turnout. The legs rotate outward from the hip socket, creating the distinctive look of the ballet dancer's feet and legs. Dancers often attempt to increase the look of their turnout by rotating the knee or ankle, or rolling the foot inward, but when they do, they run the risk of serious injury.

Find *your* turnout by placing your heels together, toes apart, in first position (a V shape) and do a *demi-plié*. If your knees are "over your toes" (in alignment, that is) that's the degree of your turnout. Adult beginners are often discouraged because their feet aren't in a straight line (perfect turnout), the way a performer's feet may appear to the audience. Naturally perfect turnout is rare, even for the professional. That's why training starts so early and requires so much practice and patience. Can adults increase their turnout? Yes, but don't expect perfection.

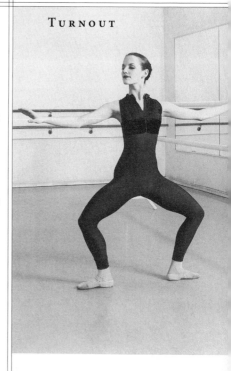

LEARNING COORDINATION: THE FOUR QUADRANTS

Adult beginners have to learn to be aware of, and to control, their extremities. Even the most coordinated and athletic adults find their hands and feet seem to have minds of their own. Their hands clutch, their arms drift up, their feet flex, all on their own. Try to imagine your body divided into four quadrants, vertically into left and right, horizontally at the hip socket. It may help you develop the control you'll need to learn ballet (it may even improve your tennis game, too).

BALLET ETIQUETTE

Ballet is indeed a world of its own. There are certain things that are just not done in a ballet class. Here's what's acceptable and what's not:

♦ Some adults may think of ballet as another adult education activity to take up, one in which they can enjoy a spirited give and take with the teacher, where they contribute ideas, and where their advice is respected and their life experiences valued.

But ballet is not an adult education class. It is different from any other class you may take, truly a throwback to another era. This means that in ballet class, the teacher conducts the class, the student is expected to follow, and unsolicited questions and witty repartee are out of place. Students do not chat or whisper with each other, or with the pianist, in ballet class.

Your teacher is the master or mistress (and these are the correct terms, just as in professional ballet companies), and even though you are not a professional, your teacher is, and adherence to the etiquette of ballet is part of the professionalism that surrounds the class.

• If you don't like a particular combination, you should still be willing to give it a try. Your teacher is giving you a combination that suits his or her pedagogical purposes (even if it doesn't seem logical or aesthetically pleasing to you). Remember that in class you have an obligation to do what the teacher asks of you, assuming you have no physical limitations.

If you absolutely don't want to, of course, you don't have to, but then you shouldn't be in class.

How best to handle it? Don't argue with the teacher or draw attention to yourself; don't make an issue of it. Instead, make your apologies, thank the teacher, take your stuff and leave. There's a discipline involved in ballet and this is part of it.

• Asking the teacher to explain something that is unclear to you is usually fine, but as a rule of thumb, if the question relates only to a problem you're having, it's better to see the teacher after class or make an appointment for a private lesson, if possible.

However, if other students are experiencing the same difficulty, it's perfectly appropriate to bring it up in class, and your teacher should be glad to address the issue by making general corrections and perhaps giving combinations that illustrate and reinforce the correction. You will also have the opportunity to ask questions and get individual attention when the teacher walks around the studio.

We have heard stories that teachers are not always gracious in responding to questions; indeed, some may seem condescending or even insulting. You needn't put up with that. Your ultimate weapon: Don't go back to that class and make your dissatisfaction known to the administration.

• In ballet class, students don't talk among themselves, and they usually don't leave the room unless permission is requested (yes, we mean it). If you have to leave for an emergency, it's not necessary, but simply more polite to catch the teacher's eye.

• If you need to leave class a bit early—to pick up your child, to catch a train—it's a courtesy to let your teacher know beforehand. Teachers are human, and they can get insulted if you leave abruptly without notice. It's good form to wait for an appropriate break before you leave: Don't dash out in the middle of a combination, for example. If it bothers the teacher to have a student slip out early, but your schedule demands it, don't take the class.

• If you come late to class, try not to arrive later than *rond de jambe* at the barre. This is for your own good; your body needs a sufficient warm-up. If you arrive late for class and the studio door is open, try to catch the teacher's eye as you slip in (do a few *pliés* to get warmed up before you pick up the class's combination). Most teachers are understanding about adult latecomers. A teacher who is not will usually close the door.

• Learn how to "space yourself" in class. This means don't get in other students' space. No matter how crowded the class, you need enough space to work full-out, and you should give others the same courtesy. There may be times when classes are so crowded that students have to alternate doing certain exercises, such as *grand battement.* For your own safety, stay out of people's way!

• If the class is divided into groups for center work, is it polite to practice along with another group? Only if you stay in the back, out of the way. As long as you work behind someone, so the teacher's attention isn't distracted from the working group, it's usually not a problem. But when in doubt, ask your teacher.

• In every class, there are always a number of students, who, for whatever reasons, are not comfortable dancing in center. It's not good form to remove yourself from your group, sit down, and watch the others. This is not a spectator sport; you are not learning to be an audience. Your teacher may be more understanding than we are and allow you to watch until you are comfortable participating. Take your cue from the teacher; if he or she insists that you try—and you don't want to—find another teacher.

What is generally acceptable: You can *stand* with the nondancing group; you can mark the steps as best you can with your group; or you can leave the class, nodding to the teacher as you go.

If center work truly throws you, your school may have a barre-only rate, which allows you to pay only for the barre portion of the class; ask about it (students who take barre-only are often more advanced dancers who want to do a barre as a warm-up and then move on to rehearsal). It does exist in many schools.

◆ In ballet, certain steps are known as "traveling steps"; these move you across the floor from one point to another. But what do you do if you tend to "travel" more quickly—meaning you jump farther—than other members of your class? If that's the case, go first. Or, go last. Just don't position yourself in the middle of the group, where you're likely to step on someone.

◆ In the dressing room: Some adults may regard dressing-room time as a social occasion, a chance to be in the company of other adults, away from professional matters, an occasion to discuss important stuff like clothes, shoes, or haircuts. This is not to say that many adult friendships haven't been made in ballet class, but the ballet dressing room, which can get overcrowded, is a place to get dressed, not to socialize. There's also an appropriate "distance" that should be maintained when people are dressing and undressing. Again, it's a courtesy.

◆ More dressing room rules: Don't monopolize the mirror or the shower in the dressing room (everyone else is in a hurry, too). Don't contribute to the mess, even if the dressing room is not as pristine as the powder room at Tiffany's. Try to be careful about edibles in the dressing room, and paper, water, or powder on the floor. Clean up after yourself when you leave. Be careful about leaving anything behind, too. It probably won't be there when you remember it.

◆ Guests in class: Teachers seldom object. This is a performing art, remember? Some adults in the class, however, may not feel ready even for an audience of one or two. If you feel uncomfortable about having people watch, tell your teacher. Your feelings are perfectly valid and should be respected.

ACCEPTING CORRECTIONS

How corrections are made and accepted by adult beginners may depend on the sensitivity of the teacher. One method teachers employ is to observe new students for a class or two, giving minimal corrections (some, so the students don't feel ignored), but letting them get comfortable and seeing how they manage on their own. "Students absorb corrections at their own speed and level, so I wait till I have a sense of how to work with them and how much they can handle," a Joffrey School faculty member explains. "If a student seems needy, for instance, I may try to give more."

Until a student absorbs correction, the teacher can't move on. For example, one Joffrey School adult beginner had a habit of twisting her body in *arabesque*. Before she advances, she must learn not to look at the leg behind her (which throws off her placement).

♦ Children in class can be distracting. There are times, however, when an adult will have no choice (we've both been in this position so we know whereof we speak). Be understanding; you may be in the same spot someday. If you have to bring your toddler, make sure he or she has something to play with. Quietly.

CORRECTIONS VERSUS CRITICISM

Dancers and aspiring professionals are used to receiving constant corrections from their teachers, from their choreographers, and from their directors—and they thrive on it. We hope you'll learn to accept correction as well, although this can be difficult for some adult beginners who don't understand the difference between correction and criticism, at first.

In the ballet class, the teacher's job is to watch and correct students as needed; the teacher's expertise is what you're paying for. Plus, in its own way, a correction can be a compliment: It implies that the teacher feels you are capable of improvement. "I get very upset when the class is so big that the teacher doesn't have time to see what I'm doing wrong," one adult beginner told us. "I'm here to be taught—and corrected!"

Almost constantly throughout the class, the teacher will make corrections aloud, sometimes directed at a specific student, other times to the class at large. Abby, a Joffrey Ballet School student, says she automatically reacts to *all* the verbal corrections her teacher calls out, whether directed at her or not. "I consider them cues to check my own position," she explains. "When the teacher calls out 'pull up, Karen' or 'heel forward, Rich,' I pull up and check my heels, too." In fact, the teacher may very well intend her corrections to work that way. Chances are, Karen wasn't the only student in the class who needed to pull up, nor Rich the only one with a sickled foot.

Corrections tend to be the same from basic ballet to the advanced, even professional level, and it's important not to be surprised (or discouraged) if you hear the same admonishments over and over again: "Shoulders down, point your foot, pull up, don't sit in the hip, square yourself off." The body doesn't do these movements naturally; it has to be constantly reminded.

Learning ballet is not so much like learning a foreign language as it is teaching your body a foreign language and bypassing your brain. Intellectually, adults often understand exactly what they're supposed to do, but their bodies may not be able to retain the physical vocabulary or corrections. But at some point, they hear the command and their bodies automatically respond. One adult student finally "got it" after two years. She internalized the concepts of *en dehors* and *en dedans* and began to do *pirouettes* correctly. This may not be possible for all adults—but as long as you're willing to come to class on a regular basis and take correction, it can happen. As your body learns the language, it will start to respond.

There are isolated instances when a teacher's corrections seem to have an edge. Teachers are human; some can be sarcastic, some impatient. Students can be oversensitive, as well. If you are the target of a correction that doesn't sound right, don't take it seriously or personally, unless it's repeated. Then, don't take it at all!

Alignment means having all the body parts in the right relationship to the whole; not only is this safest, it feels best. Plus, once learned, alignment cues have a way of carrying over into your daily life.

PROPER POSTURE

"Posture" is really a layperson's term. It's what your mother had in mind when she told you, "Stand up straight" or, "Don't hunch your shoulders," but it's really not a dancer's concept. Still, by the time they reach their teens, young dancers do hold themselves erect in that beautiful and distinctive way most people relate to "good posture."

As you attend ballet classes, the way you stand, walk, and move (all generally thought of as posture) will improve. As it does, you'll see it's not a matter of "keeping your back straight" (impossible, the back has a natural curve) or "holding your shoulders down" (how *do* you do that?) but of gaining better awareness and understanding of how your body works, what's going on inside it, and, most important, of pulling up.

Ballet consists of movements that may not be as unnatural as they seem (as Joffrey School teacher Liz D'Anna pointed out, they can be compared to more mundane actions). Once you accept that fact, we can use a "natural" placement of the body to describe proper ballet posture.

In essence, ballet posture is your normal, natural body placement with the addition of the pulling-up concept (and a few other touches). It's what takes an everyday body and makes it a dancer's body. Ballet posture tones the stomach muscles, lengthens the look of the torso, and straightens the upper back.

Start by standing up straight. In ballet, standing straight means just that: The pelvis is tilted neither forward or backward. For example, if you exaggerate the natural curve of the back, it's wrong; if you "tuck" your pelvis, it's wrong. A pelvic tilt changes the curve of your spine and prevents you from moving, and anything that hinders your ability to move, hinders your ability to dance.

With ballet posture, the neck is long. The chin is level (neither tucked in nor thrust out). Your stomach is pulled in; your body pulled up, your shoulders are pulled back and down. If you concentrate on the latter, it should also help alleviate tension across the back and neck, a major knotting place. Other considerations: Your hips are square; facing straight ahead. Your weight is distributed evenly on your legs (resting on one leg thrusts one hip out—which you don't want).

To help you imagine this posture, one teacher uses the image of a stack of spools of thread. If one spool isn't properly in place, the entire stack is out of alignment and may topple. In ballet, if anything is improperly placed, you can't stand up straight. And if you can't stand up straight, you can't dance.

Most adult classes are ongoing. The good news is that you can start at any time and you can take as many or as few classes as you're able. Multiply this by as many people who are taking the class and the result is a different mix of students, of varying degrees of experience, every day. In every Joffrey School adult beginner class, for example, there will be new students, some who have studied before, some who haven't. The challenge for the teacher who is trying to present material systematically is to keep the experienced students interested and not lose the newcomers. This means that inevitably, absolute beginners are going to have to pick up some basics on their own.

Unless you attend the first class, you probably won't be taught the five positions of the feet. So here they are:

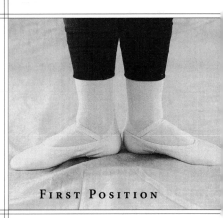

FIRST POSITION

First position:
Put your heels together, with your toes facing out. Your feet make a V. Your knees are straight and all your toes are on the floor.

BALLET-FIT TIP

Try not to roll inward or outward, which can happen in first position when you try to work with more turnout than you have. How wide a V you make depends on your turnout so start with less—a small V—and gradually open it.

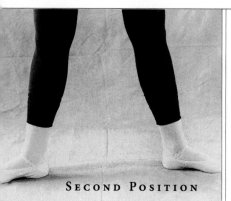

SECOND POSITION

Second position:

Second is the same as first position but with your feet apart, your knees aligned with your toes, and your back straight.

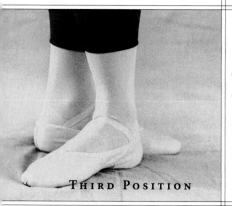

THIRD POSITION

Third position:

The feet are partly crossed. The heel of the front foot rests near the arch of the back foot.

Fifth position: (No, this is not a mistake. It's just easier to describe fifth before fourth): In fifth, your feet are completely crossed. The heel of the front foot rests against the toe of the back foot.

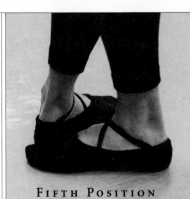

FIFTH POSITION

BALLET-FIT TIP

Don't worry if your feet are not necessarily together or "closed." A space between the toes of the front foot and the heel of the back foot is perfectly acceptable and, for adult beginners, usual. If you had perfect turnout, you could close your fifth. If you try to close without perfect turnout, you'll place too much stress on your knees and ankles.

Fourth position: It's the same as fifth, with the width of one of your own feet between the front foot and the back foot.

BALLET-FIT TIP

Put your feet in fifth position. Move the front foot forward so there's a space between the two feet (it's just like the relationship between first and second). Fourth is often the last position that teachers use because it's so hard to keep your hips square.

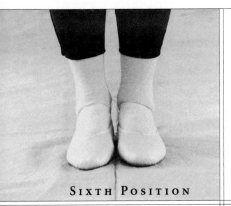

Sixth position (and you thought there were only five): Children and absolute beginners are sometimes taught in sixth position, with the feet parallel, facing front.

BALLET-FIT TIP

At the Joffrey School, we call this position what it is—feet parallel—but at some schools it's known as sixth position.

For the first two classes, you'll probably use only two of the five basic positions: first position and second. Then you'll progress to fifth, and lastly to fourth. Where's third? Again, at the Joffrey School, we don't use third because it's not used on stage.

All About Arms

Arms are hard to discuss because we feel negative about them, at least in terms of the way they're sometimes taught in ballet class. Although we dance with our arms as well as our legs, we really believe that keeping the arms simple is what best serves the adult beginner, both from an aesthetic and a fitness point of view. Beginners haven't developed the strength, control, or aesthetic sensibility to use *port de bras* in an artistic way. Or, the coordination: Arms can be difficult because the upper arm is rotating outward while the forearm is rotating inward, all of which means it's often hard enough to learn the legs without complicating things by adding arms. Still, some teachers do add arms because you've got to learn them sooner or later—and because they do add to the feeling of dance. *Always follow your teacher; it's the teacher who choreographs the arms in ballet class.*

We find, however, that the best approach for adult beginners is to get the arms out of the way: Put your hands on your waist or shoulders to start with, then in second position for most of the class (holding your arms *à la seconde* actually helps firm and develop the arm muscles almost without your realizing it). As you progress, your teacher should introduce simple arms to accompany your combinations. Make sure that you use the muscles in your back (the lattisimus dorsi) and all the shoulder blade muscles (scapular stabilizers) to control your arms, so your shoulders stay calm (shoulders tend to tense and creep up to your ears) and your neck stays long. As for your hands, hold your fingers naturally (don't clench or curl), and make sure your thumbs don't stick up.

Below, some additional pointers:

♦ In second position, don't allow your arm to bend (bent elbows resemble broken wings) or drift forward or backward, which can pull your shoulder out of alignment.

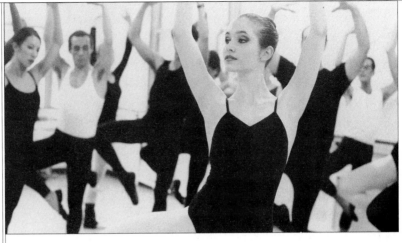

Arms are as much a part of ballet as feet. En haut seems to be everyone's favorite position in class.

◆ Don't break the line of the arm at the wrist. Instead, the arm should appear to be one piece, from the shoulders to the tips of the fingers—like a pipe cleaner!

◆ As we said earlier, arms are choreographed, which means it's up to your teacher to call for different arm movements to accompany different steps. In general, though, the arms usually go up (*en haut*) when your foot is in the front, *à la seconde,* when your foot is to the side, and *arabesque* arms (straight in front at shoulder level or slanted slightly upward in line with the nose) when your foot is in the back. In *relevé* and *sous-sus,* the arms usually go *en haut;* with *frappés, en bas.* Try to avoid getting into the habit of automatic arm movements, such as instinctively raising your arms *en haut* in fifth *relevé.* Unless your teacher calls for it, don't assume.

Every teacher, at the Joffrey School and elsewhere, has his or her own way of using the arms. Beauty is in the eye of the beholder and it's up to your teacher to determine the aesthetics of the arms in class.

PREPARATIONS AND PROPER FINISHES

Preparations and finishes are as much a part of ballet as accents are to French. Preparations allow you to get ready, or "in position" (with your weight over your standing leg, for example), for difficult steps such as *rond de jambe* or *frappés*. Proper finishes such as *demi-plié*, after you complete one side of the barre and turn to the other, add polish and are a graceful completion to the combination. Both are integral parts of ballet class, not to be ignored or forgotten.

In *frappé*, the traditional preparation is a simple *tendu* to the side, although sometimes teachers precede *frappés* with flexing movements, half-point exercises or other variations. Since *frappés* are something of a ballet oddity (they're the only exercise that's done with a flexed foot rather than a pointed one), we have to admit that liberties are taken here.

Rond de jambe calls for a two-part preparation: a *plié* and *tendu* front, all in one movement; then as you straighten your leg, a *tendu* to the side. This preparation opens the hip and helps "set you up."

In the adult classes at the Joffrey, we also ask for a simple preparation with the arms. This is done for every exercise, usually to four counts of music. You listen for the first two counts; on the next two, the arm extends to the front, then to the side (*à la seconde*).

After you complete a combination, traditionally, you end in a *demi-plié*, arms *en bas*. If you finish your combination in a *relevé*, and then turn to the other side, you release into a *demi-plié*, then straighten, arms *en bas*, as well. Always. This finishing *demi-plié* is not a perfunctory movement, a quick bob or a half-hearted bent knee, but a deep and elastic *demi-plié* using all your muscles, as the music trails off. And, like a preparation, it's not an extra or afterthought, but one of the touches that lend polish to your class per-

---

BALLET-FIT TIP

When you finish a combination of any kind, you do a *demi-plié* and straighten up with your arm *en bas*—and don't move till the music stops. It's a real *demi-plié*, too—don't make it an afterthought—which not only finishes the combination in an appropriate way but relieves tension in the legs and keeps you from getting stiff.

---

formance. Also, when you complete a combination and "turn to the other side," you always turn toward the barre, not away from it. Why? It's considered good manners—another part of ballet tradition!

They say an audience always remembers the last thing they see, so even if you bungle the combination or forget the sequence halfway through, try to wind up with a proper ballet finish. Wait until the music is completely through. Your feet should be in the final position of the completed exercise (usually fifth or first), your arms gracefully curved *en bas,* your head looking over the outside shoulder. Even if it's not required, you'll look very professional. And when everyone in the adult class does it, it looks like a ballet class should.

Beginner Head Movements

In class you may see some students coordinating their head movements with their arms; it looks as if they know what they're doing and you may want to emulate them, but keep in mind, they may not.

On the whole, in ballet, the head does follow the arms. When the arm is down, the head is slightly lowered; when the arms are to the side, the head looks to the side, over the shoulder. If your teacher hasn't given your class specific instructions regarding head movements as yet, keep your head to the front or to the side (so you can see yourself in the mirror and self-correct if need be). And remember that until your teacher feels you are ready for head movements, what looks pretty in your imagination may look fussy to your teacher. Think twice before emulating anything you may have seen in more advanced classes or on stage. Which brings us to . . .

Affectations to Avoid

Once you're into ballet both as an art and as an exercise, you may want to do more. At the very least, you'll want to attend more performances or watch ballet on video or perhaps try a more advanced class. And you'll see lots of things you may be tempted to

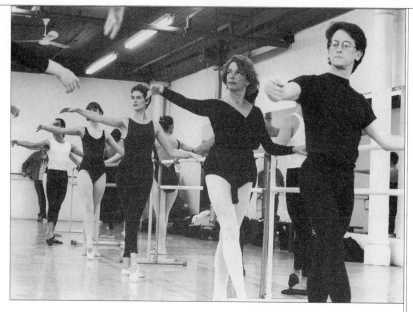

Best thing for arms is keep it simple. Don't be tempted to try things you've seen on stage or on tape. These students working on perfecting their à la seconde.

try, which is what inspired this section. An extra flutter of the hands or flourish of the wrist. An exaggerated head movement or "flowery," overly "expressive" *port de bras*. Personal stylizations or "creative" variations of the combination that the teacher has not asked for. Nice? Not really. All of these fall under the heading of "affectations to avoid" and are not appropriate or attractive in an adult beginner class.

At the Joffrey Ballet School, as at many other professional schools, the look is clean and classic, and students are expected to follow the teacher's choreography without embellishment. The exception: If you have a teacher who was trained that way and wants you to follow her, then do it. Your teacher is always right.

In addition, as we suggested earlier, we don't recommend emulating the professional dancers you've seen on tape or in professional classes (or even on stage) in your beginner class. Often professional dancers develop habits that were not taught and that may even be technically incorrect. They may, for example, begin a *plié* before a *tendu* is complete. Or they may lift their heels slightly in *demi-plié* or land a jump without putting their heels down. We can't chide a working professional, but she probably knows better, and so should you. You may be familiar enough with the basics to notice and experiment with nuance, but some of your beginner classmates won't be. And, at that point, it's their class, not yours.

Some teachers are tolerant of advanced or professional dancers doing their own versions of combinations in class, or even adding their own more complex *port de bras,* all to the great confusion of those standing around them. In an adult beginner class, this is inconsiderate at best and a distraction and disservice to those who belong in the class. Some teachers may be reluctant to correct those students or even remind them that they are guests in your class. If so, learn to ignore their behavior, and don't follow them. If you wish to watch and learn from advanced students, take their class or ask permission to observe.

Ballet classes on videotape differ from each other as much or as little as any other ballet class. You may learn a great deal or you might pick up some unusual habits. If a video teacher is similar in method and approach to your teacher, you can't help but benefit from the extra work. If their styles are incompatible, however, keep searching for another tape or keep your live class separate from your video class.

Rule of thumb: Don't add anything that your teacher hasn't.

What to Do When You're Feeling Confident

So what can you do in class when you're feeling confident? Is it a faux pas to ask your teacher to introduce a new step that you've seen on tape or in performance? Not at all. Teachers should respond graciously, whether the answer is "yes" or "no," but bear in mind that his or her obligation is to teach to the level of the class. If you're the only student who could possibly absorb the new work (which is called "vocabulary"), your teacher may work with you briefly after class or refer you to another class or even ask a more advanced student to demonstrate the step for you.

But there are also ways a teacher can introduce new vocabulary, making it accessible to all members of your class. You needn't be shy about asking, as long as you realize that it is not always possible to accommodate the emerging advanced beginner without antagonizing the rest of the class.

What you can do without arousing the jealousy or competitive spirit of your peers is to make the class harder for yourself. Below are some suggestions which are generally acceptable in an adult beginner class (in fact, your teacher may even routinely offer the class the option to perform a movement in *relevé* instead of flat, for those students who wish to challenge themselves):

◆ Vary a combination by doing part of it in *relevé,* instead of flat. Try doing your *passés* or *développés* in *relevé.*

◆ Test your balance from time to time by removing your hand from the barre during *frappé,* for example, or anytime at the barre, especially when one leg is off the floor.

◆ Do the center combinations with each group (working behind so as not to get in the way or appear to demand extra attention).

◆ Add beats to jumps, do "double" *frappés,* do the men's combinations, try multiple *pirouettes,* hold your balances longer. But be prepared for the possibility of some negative reactions from some of your classmates. Ballet, even at the adult beginner level, can get competitive!

◆ The ultimate: Speak to your teacher about starting *pointe* work. If you're strong, it may be an option!

Counting Music

How much does the adult beginner have to know about music? Does the music in ballet class tell you anything about the steps? Not really. But the more you know, the greater your enjoyment of class, because one art enhances the other. Still, in order to count the music in ballet class, all you really have to know is how to count to eight. Period.

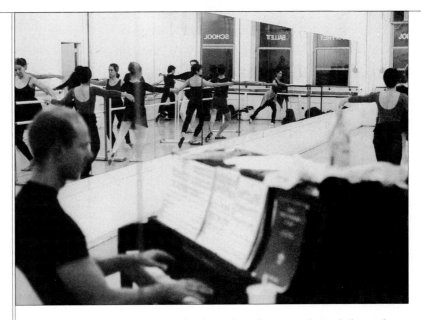

Not every school or studio can provide live accompaniment. There are excellent audiotapes and CD's available for studio use that you can also use at home.

In music, there is also the beat (or the count), and the upbeat (this is the part that you count as "and"). In ballet class, sometimes the accent is on the beat; sometimes it's on the upbeat (most people can actually hear the difference; the beat is louder). What if you can't hear the difference? Don't worry. Your teacher will tell you where the accent is. For example, for *grands battements* or *dégagés,* the accent may be on the closing. For *rond de jambe,* the accent is on the direction you're going in. If you're going front (*en dehors*), your foot goes forward on the count.

If you don't quite get this, at some point your body probably will. And if your teacher is at all interested in the musical aspect of the class, he or she will be articulating it for you. Some teachers, of course, may not have musical training; they don't have to be able to articulate it, they just feel it. And some pianists are so accomplished that you may feel it, too, whether you know it or not.

MEN IN TIGHTS

Because guys are always outnumbered by girls, they are cherished in class. Really. In fact, at the Joffrey School, we love having men in class—they bring a different dimension because they are used to moving in a different way (plus they don't have the same ballet fantasy that so many women have, as a carryover from their childhood). Specifically, the articulation of a man's feet and hands isn't the same as a woman's; men point their feet differently; and generally their movements are sports-oriented rather than dance-oriented (men often have muscles that have developed as a result of sports, that in fact conflict with their movements in class).

In the ballet school or studio, men are always treated with great respect in the hopes that they will stay (the fact is, sometimes men don't last in class; they don't seem to have the patience to stick it out—and ballet is a long process!). Because of the general shortage of male dancers, it's even possible for a man to begin a professional career at a much later age than a woman. Ron is one talented student we recall who originally came to the Joffrey School's adult beginner classes when in his late twenties—traditionally far too late to begin a career. He advanced quickly, eventually got a schol-

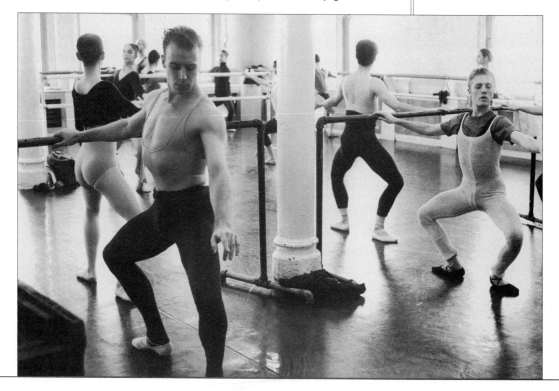

arship, and is now completing his training with a professional company. Granted, he's an exception, but it does happen.

But most men come to adult ballet with nonprofessional goals in mind. Often they're involved in other sports—basketball or boxing, for instance, and they find that ballet training helps them move. Men who are into weight lifting say it's one of the most effective ways to develop flexibility and stretch—neglected in weight training and important especially if you're getting overly muscled. In fact, men find ballet training useful for all kinds of sports, from tennis to baseball to football.

Some male athletes, however, may find ballet class a bit daunting at first. It seems so different from the sports they're used to. With most sports a little knowledge goes a long way (you develop a certain amount of expertise, you can play—at some level). But with ballet, there's more to learn, and it seems so foreign. Every guy has dribbled a basketball at some point in his life, every guy has bent his knees to ski or play tennis, but not every guy knows he's doing *pliés!* Too, the muscles men develop as a result of sports may conflict with their turnout in class, so it can be a challenge.

Still, when it clicks, it clicks, and the guys say they find ballet as rewarding as the women (in fact, when one man finally "got" the barre, he said it was like having a religious experience!).

Many men in class are actors; ballet is simply part of their stage training. Or musicians. Jonathan works in finance. Scott drives a truck. Rich works for his local power-supply company. After he got seriously involved with ballroom dancing, he was advised to take up ballet.

The fact is, men get many of the same benefits from ballet class that women do. It's a great way to get in touch with your body, slim down, develop strength where you need it (your upper body, your legs, your torso).

In the Joffrey Ballet School's adult classes, we find that men often come for the athletics and stay for the aesthetics. They discover a whole new world.

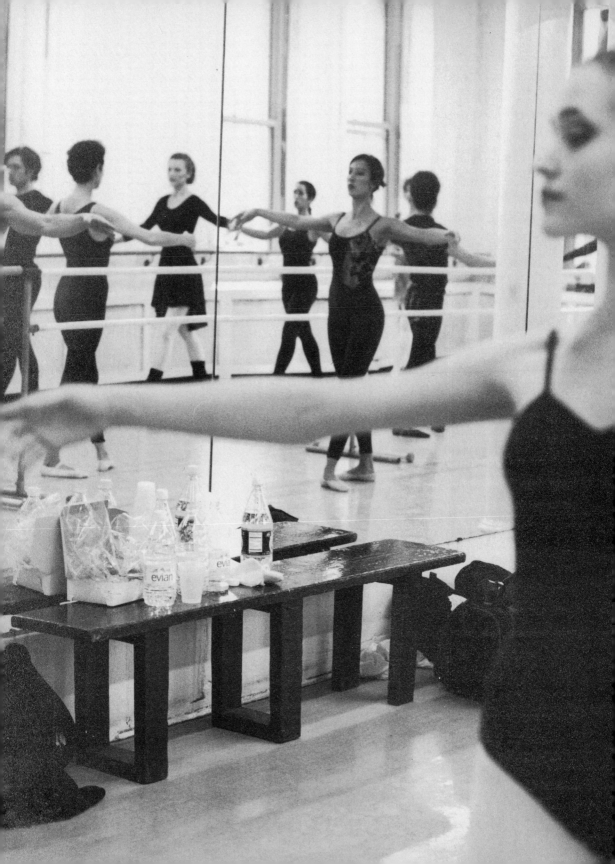

6

*B*asic Barre and Center

e⁓

NOW YOU'VE GOT THE etiquette and language of the ballet class; you've learned something of the procedures; you know about its fitness benefits; you may even have bought shoes and a leotard. You've got the words; now what about the actions?

Ballet is learned by imitation and repetition. When children take ballet classes, they don't analyze and they don't understand description, except on the simplest levels (they do understand fanciful descriptions along the lines of "imagine you're an icicle" when doing *relevé*). Most children don't have enough vocabulary or experience to learn in ways other than observing, following and repeating, and having their arms, legs, tummies, and backs pushed and coaxed until they can feel the positions and re-create those feelings on command.

Adults learn that way, too, but they also can relate what they're learning, seeing, and feeling in class to a lifetime of other experiences. Exercisers are acquainted with their muscles. Theatergoers have been exposed to ballet movement. Travelers use other languages. Film buffs—and anyone who watches TV—hear more and more classical music, which is regularly used in movie soundtracks and even as background in TV commercials. Drivers are comfortable with directionality. Everyone uses a mirror.

Banishing Ballet-Speak

Here, we've tried to analyze and break down basic beginner ballet vocabulary in order to present it in the most accessible way. We've attempted to banish "ballet-speak," but since dancers, like all professionals, have a proprietary interest in having their own language, with jargon that triggers different images, we'll try to explain some of it, too. Keep in mind that one image may not work for you, but another word or phrase might. That's the advantage of learning by repetition. Over the course of many months, the movement is presented and described in many different ways, one of which (we hope) will click.

In putting together this chapter, we've talked about whether we are venturing into the realm of "technique," which refers to something very special to the professional dancer. Our conclusion: not at all. That's because technique, as understood by the dancer (or the serious student of ballet), has its own special meaning; it hardly carries the same connotations or expectations for the adult ballet student. Rather, what we are offering are definitions in easy-to-understand English and practical pointers on achieving correct form, plus how-to's, hints, and other verbal cues that have worked and worked well for other adult ballet students. Our goal is to make it easier for you to reap the many benefits and pleasures of your adult class, and, we hope, bring you one step closer to "getting it right."

With all of this in mind, as you approach the barre, we want you to feel strong and to feel confident. Make your movements definite, not tentative; make your mistakes; make them with courage and conviction. And now, let's go to the barre. . . .

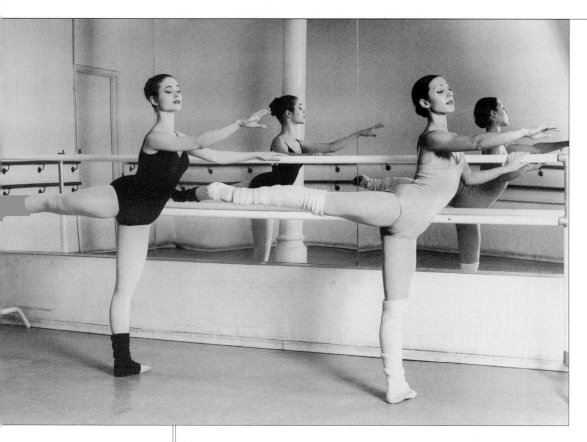

ARABESQUE

The term *arabesque* can refer to both a position and a direction. As a position, *arabesque* means any action or extension of a straight leg to the back (bent legs are *attitude*). But your teacher may use the word as a direction, meaning to the back, as in *tendu arabesque* for a *tendu* back.

CAMBRÉ

Cambré means "arched" and refers to the stretches and bends of the upper body that start the barre, warming up your body's muscles, getting you to breathe deeply, opening your lungs.

When you *cambré* or bend forward, the key thing is to work from the hip joint rather than the waist. We can't emphasize this strongly enough! As you bend forward, for example, try to be conscious of pulling up and out of your hips (think of reaching *forward* with your chest—not bending down to pick up a hairpin). You should feel the stretch in your hamstrings (the muscle in the back of the thigh).

When you're doing *cambrés,* the teacher may surprise you by asking for a *grand port de bras* as part of the *cambré* combination. If so, be prepared: the *grand port de bras* is just a continuous, circular *cambré*—first forward, then to the side, then back and to the side (and usually reversed)—a smooth, flowing, circular movement of the upper body.

If you've never seen a *grand port de bras* before in class, look around you, watch the other students out of the corner of your eye, and give it a try. It only looks dramatic: it's really a very nice stretch of the torso and not all that different from what you've been doing in simple *port de bras,* except that it's all in one action. Note, too, that it goes *en dehors* and *en dedans* (from front to back and then reversed).

As you do your *port de bras,* your head should move in harmony with your arm, gracefully and subtly following its movements. Keep your fingers relaxed (don't stick your thumb out), your wrist firm, and your hand curved.

Don't twist your body (use both shoulders when you *cambré* back).

Don't stick your tummy out when you *cambré* back.

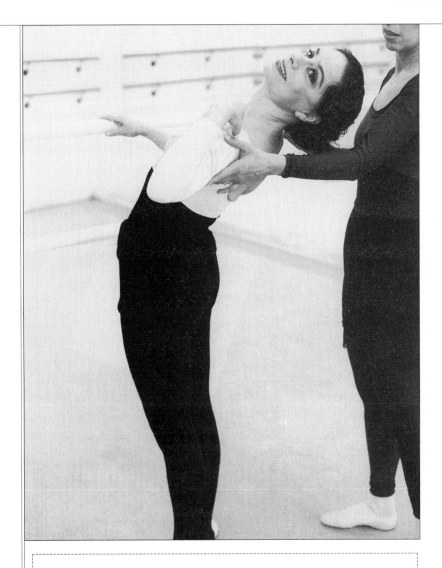

How do you know how far away from the barre to stand? Place your arms in second position. Your inside hand should rest lightly on the barre. If your elbow rests on the barre, you're too close, which will distort your body line, crowding your arm and hunching your shoulder. If you have to reach for the barre, you're too far away. Not only will this pull your body out of alignment but you won't have the support you need.

PLIÉS

You know what a *plié* is (you probably knew it without knowing that you know it!). That's because *pliés* are one of the most widely known of all ballet movements. Many a nonballet workout, in fact, includes *pliés* because of their leg strengthening and firming benefits, especially to the inner thigh, which always seems to be the part of the body that adult students dislike the most.

Not only do *pliés* work the inner thigh, they also work the abdominals. After a while, if you do enough *pliés,* while we won't guarantee a perfect body (or perfect inner thighs), you will notice a difference.

As for what they are, *grands pliés* can best be described as a ballet version of a deep knee bend. *Demi-pliés* are not so deep.

The first thing the adult ballet student has to understand is that any *plié* is an outward motion, not a downward one (this sometimes comes as a surprise to beginners). But throughout the action of the *plié, grand* or *demi,* and in all of the positions, the body stays lifted and long, the knees face outward (not forward) so that the dancer always feels tall, even though he or she is giving the impression of moving downward.

At the barre, we like to start with *demi-pliés* in second (this is a personal idiosyncrasy; most teachers start in first position). By starting in second, beginners are introduced to the concept of keeping their heels down in *plié. Pliés* then are performed in all the positions, although in absolute beginner classes, *pliés* in fourth posi-

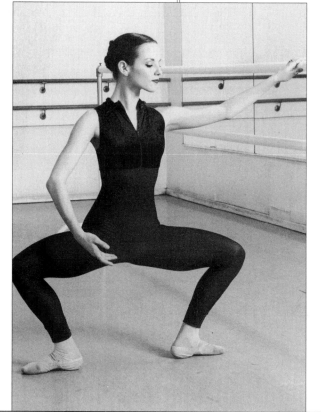

SOME DON'TS

Don't turn your toes out too much (you'll twist your knees).

Don't *plié* with your knees forward.

Don't let your backside stick out (check yourself in the mirror).

Don't round your back by bending forward at the waist.

THE TURNOUT

When you attend a ballet performance you can't help noticing the turnout. So when you take your place at the barre for the first time and are asked to assume first position, you may be tempted to put your heels together with your toes outward at a 180-degree angle. It'll look like a straight line, but if you're like most people, you'll fall over.

While everyone has natural turnout from the hips, it's the rare person who has the degree of rotation in the hip that is a must for the performing dancer. Don't try to augment your natural turnout by pushing your feet outward or twisting your knees or ankles. If you don't have the flexibility and strength from the hips, your arches may roll in (see page 100); you could strain your ankles, knees, or back. Keep your feet in a fifth, first, or second position without straining and you'll do fine.

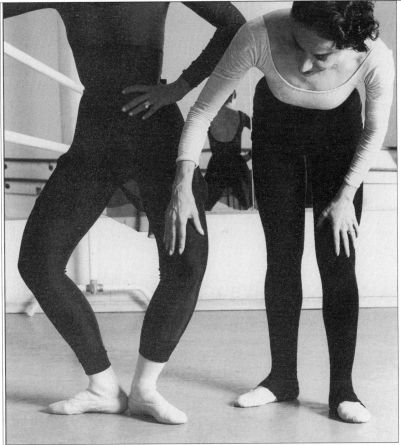

tion may be omitted because they require more turnout than many students have at that point. Remember that your school, like the Joffrey School, may not use third position, which all too often looks like a sloppy fifth position. On the other hand, your school may substitute third position for fifth position in its adult classes, since it is generally less stressful.

Beginners often *plié* "backside first," which creates the look of sticking your seat out. To avoid this, keep your back absolutely straight. You may also hear your teacher warn you against "sitting in your *plié*" or tell you to "keep your knees active." This just means keep moving! Just as a *plié* is an outward motion, it's also a continuous one. When you get to the bottom of the *plié*, immediately start moving upward: don't hold. All *pliés* are movements, not poses. How far should your knees bend in *demi-plié*? Stretch your inner thighs and go as far as you can without lifting the heels.

Grand plié is deeper, but the rules still apply. It, too, is a outward, continuous motion. Start with your *demi-plié* and continue the movement by lifting your heels just barely, till you reach what's called "the bottom of your *plié*." That means as low as you can (the heels should never be as high as they are in *relevé*). In second position, though, your heels *never* lift, so your *grand plié* will not be as deep. In all positions, your knees stay over your toes, your thighs are stretching, your back is straight. Older dancers or anyone with knee problems should think twice about *grands pliés,* and skip them if they hurt.

Arms for *pliés?* If you wish to "do your own arms," we suggest the first *port de bras,* the outside arm moving as the legs move, going from second through fifth *en bas,* through first, and opening in second, at the conclusion of the *plié.* As the arm movements correspond with the legs, you'll notice that the upper body and the lower body are doing two different things.

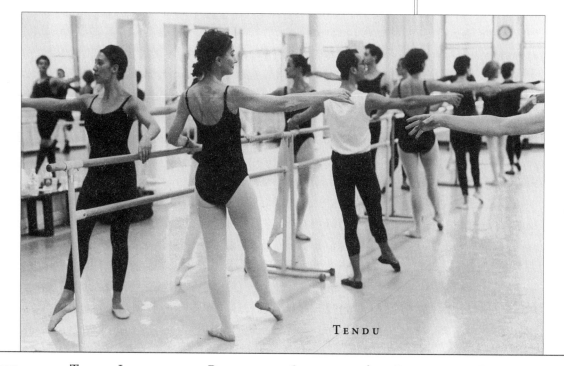

TENDU

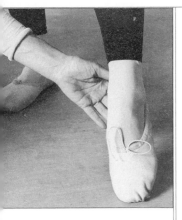

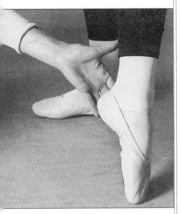

SOME DOS AND DON'TS

Watch out for floppy feet (keep the leg stretched).

Avoid sickling (keep the heels forward).

Don't let the inside of the heel drop back (again, keep the heel forward).

Keep the toe in line with the heel of the standing leg.

TENDU

Tendu is the first exercise after *pliés*. When you work slowly and deliberately in *tendu*, with focus and concentration, you set yourself up for the rest of the class—your abdominals are beginning to work, you're on your standing leg, your working leg is beginning to be stretched. In fact, we conceptualize the ballet barre as based on the *tendu*; it's the foundation of almost everything else.

Think of *tendu* as a process, not a position. The end result of the *tendu* is a pointed foot, but how you get to the pointed foot is the *tendu*, too. For ballet purposes, *tendus* warm and strengthen the foot, and they start working the hip socket to prepare the body for the weight shifts ahead. They are also low-level isolation exercises that help develop balance, work the buttocks muscles (and since you should be holding your tummy in, they work the abdominals too).

We like to think of *tendu* as a slow, systematic stretch of the leg and foot. This is accomplished by sliding the foot along the floor, until it's fully stretched, then pulling it back. The key to a beautiful *tendu* is to keep your heel forward and to "use your whole foot," a phrase you may hear your ballet teacher use. "Use your whole foot" means that as you slide your foot forward, think of your foot as articulate as a hand, and push down against the floor, feeling the floor under your entire foot, until it gradually points. When your leg and foot are fully stretched in *tendu*, only the very tip of your big toe, or possibly also your second toe, will remain on the floor.

The *tendu* is also a perfect example of a weight-shift exercise. In the starting position (first, fifth), your weight is on both feet. Then the weight shifts to the standing leg, freeing the working leg to complete the *tendu*. The weight doesn't shift back until the *tendu* is completed and you close on two feet again.

The *tendu* is an important part of ballet vocabulary. It's a strong and conscious exercise that requires a lot of energy on the part of the student. It should not be easy, but it should look it.

RELEVÉ

Relevé means to stand on tiptoes (more formally known as *demi-pointe*). Think of lifting the heels and leaving the ball of the foot flat on the floor. The back is straight, the legs are stretched and turned out from the hip socket, the heels are forward, and if all five toes are on the floor you'll have a nice, reasonably solid base of support. Related to *relevé* in fifth position is *sous-sus*. Both feet are held tight together creating a fifth position *relevé* without any space between the legs. Think of using your inner thighs to bring the legs together; properly done, the two feet brace each other.

Even little children can usually do nice *relevés*, but of course, we don't ask little children to do *relevé* on one leg. But you're not a child, and you should know that you will be asked to balance *en relevé* on one leg, as well as on two. When this happens, you just shift your weight to your standing leg, and all the same *relevé* rules apply.

Either way, if your *relevés* are wobbly and you can't "find your balance," try to consciously pull up on the ankles and focus on the ball of the foot. You have to be "high" on the *relevé*, which means your heels should be as high as they can go (imagine you're wearing four-inch stilettos), and your ankles should be in line with your toes. To center yourself, lift yourself up and out of the hip sockets—feel very long—and keep your shoulders down and relaxed.

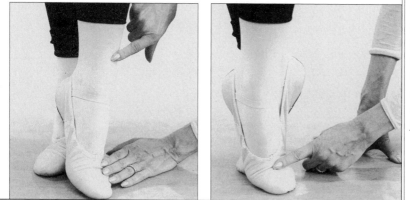

En relevé, *be careful that the ankle doesn't drop back, creating a sickled effect, and of putting too much weight on the outside of the foot (far left). All five toes should feel the floor (near left).*

We have just one more reminder here: Don't automatically throw your arms up in the air (*en haut*), unless your teacher directs you. *Relevés* are so often taught with arms *en haut* that it becomes a habit. But arms, once again, are always choreographed, so avoid doing any *ports de bras* that are not specifically given.

BALLET-FIT TIP

At the barre, you may be asked to *relevé* and do a *soutenu* turn. To do this, simply pivot, changing the front/back relationship of the feet (that's *soutenu*). It's easy: Just don't lose your turnout and think about controlling the turning movement with your inner thighs.

BATTEMENT TENDU JETÉ (A.K.A. BATTEMENT DÉGAGÉ OR BATTEMENT GLISSÉ)

Battements tendus jetés (*jeté* means "thrown") are the same as *tendus* but with a little more spring to them. And there's a brushing action. As in *tendu,* the foot slides along the floor. When the leg and foot are fully stretched in *tendu,* the foot lifts off the floor with a quick burst of energy.

Battements tendus jetés to the back can sometimes be a problem, so be especially aware of maintaining your turnout here. Also, as in any movement to the back, your hips will open up (it's impossible to stay perfectly "square" but it is an ideal to shoot for). One trick is to keep in mind that the "audience" needs to see the top of your foot, not the profile, which requires that you use your turnout. You may get lots of corrections here. It's why even in advanced classes you tend to hear the same corrections over and over again.

Related to the *battement tendu jeté* is *balançoire* or *en cloche:* The working foot brushes front, through first position and back, in a continuous movement.

SOME DOS AND DON'TS

Don't drop your heels back when you do *battement tendu jeté* to the side.

Don't bend your knees.

Do feel the stretch of the fully extended leg.

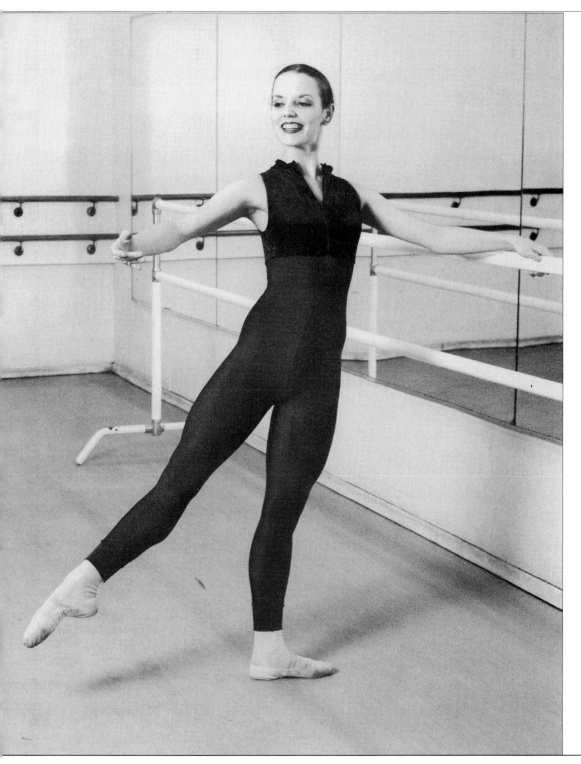

Basic Barre and Center

ROND DE JAMBE

Ronds des jambes are nothing more than *tendus* that go around in a semicircle, *en dehors* and *en dedans*, on the floor (*par terre*) and off the floor (*en l'air*). In other words, *ronds des jambes* are about turnout—getting it and holding it from the hip socket.

When you do *rond de jambe*, your working leg is the only part of your body that is moving. Your body, your hips, and your supporting leg should remain still as your working leg moves in a semicircle through first position, fourth front, second position, *arabesque* (back), returning to first position. Keep your leg straight, with only the barest contact between your foot and the floor (but there should be some contact).

If you remember to lead with the inside of the heel you'll find *rond de jambe en dedans* a bit easier than *en dehors*. Try to focus on keeping your heel forward (as if you were presenting the inside of your heel to an audience). Holding your turnout in *rond de jambe*

SOME DOS AND DON'TS

Don't turn in as you go through first position. Hit your first position every time.

Don't let the heel drop back (this means don't sickle).

Keep contact with the floor.

Keep the inside of the heel forward (or presented to the audience in every position and in every direction).

Keep both knees straight.

Keep your hips as square as possible.

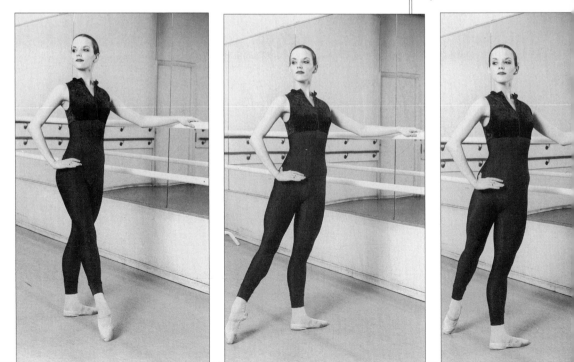

is also more difficult as your leg moves from the side to the back. This is where you have to be conscious of the rotation of your leg in the hip socket. Again, without lifting the hip or bending the knee, present the inside of your heel to the audience, and you'll be fine.

What Advanced Dancers Do and Why Not to Follow Them

We've mentioned that your foot should be in contact with the floor during *rond de jambe.* Sometimes, though, you may see more advanced students barely graze the floor. While it's not technically correct (the floor should be felt with two toes, or at least the big toe), they are working on speed. Touching the floor more firmly may slow them down.

In addition, a more advanced dancer's *rond de jambe* may not even be a complete semicircle (in other words, it won't fully reach the *tendu* front and the *tendu* back position but instead makes an elliptical pattern). This only works when your body is anatomically ready for such a variation. According to *Inside Technique,* by Valerie Grieg (a terrific book about dancer's anatomy, it's geared toward the professional, but we highly recommend it anyway), an elliptical pattern places more emphasis on the action taking place in the hip socket. While valuable for the professional or career-track dancer, the adult beginner's emphasis should be on working correctly; that is, hitting your position, front and back. We feel strongly that the adult beginner should learn what is technically correct. Rule of thumb: Always follow your teacher, not the professional dancer who is "visiting" your class.

F R A P P É

Frappés are different from everything else that's done at the barre and are often disconcerting to the adult beginner who is used to working with a pointed foot. In *frappé*, though, we bend the knee of the working leg, and we flex the working foot so it is at right angles to your leg (*coupé*). As the ball of your foot strikes the floor (front, side, or back) the only movement should be from the knee and at the ankle, as the foot goes from the flex to the point. Keeping everything turned out, of course. And therein lie the difficulties.

In class, we often joke about "fear of *frappés*," but beautifully executed *frappés* are far from an insurmountable obstacle for the adult beginner. One way to think about *frappés* is that the starting position (foot flexed in a *coupé*) is like a *demi-plié* with one leg. Be sure to return to that flexed foot in *coupé* (don't let the *coupé*

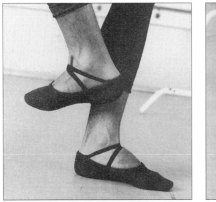
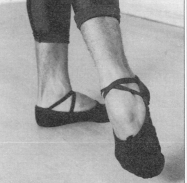
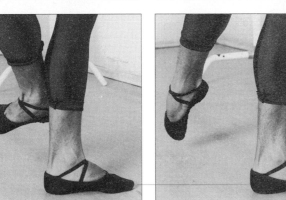

THE JOFFREY BALLET SCHOOL'S BALLET-FIT

"drop") each time. Where to place the foot in *coupé*? We like it somewhere between the ankle bone and the bottom of the calf muscle, although some teachers may place it a little lower. But the point is to keep the knee facing outward and your entire weight on your standing leg.

The *frappé* action can also be thought of as a simulated jump in first position: Visualize the flexed foot in *coupé* as half a *demi-plié* in first position. Then visualize the end of the *frappé* (after the foot strikes the floor) as the height of the jump in first position, with the leg straight in the air and the working foot *pointed*.

If this doesn't help, think of *frappés* as analogous to *battements tendus jetés*, in which the foot is brushed along the floor. The difference is that the leg starts with a bent knee rather than a straight one.

If that doesn't work, watch your teacher.

What else makes *frappés* so difficult? They're so different from everything else in class; they fall in the second half of the barre when students are beginning to tire; and they're usually done at a fairly lively tempo—they're quick (although in a beginner class, they shouldn't be too quick). If the tempo is too fast for you, remember that it's a far far better thing to do one beautiful *frappé* than three sloppy ones. And hang in there. *Frappés* can be conquered. You may even find yourself doing double *frappés* in just a matter of months.

A D A G I O

The structure of the barre is based on alternating slow and fast exercises, which is why *adagio,* a series of slow movements, usually follows *frappés* at the barre. But in addition to *adagio*'s contrast of rhythm, its slow, stretchy movements should relieve tension, as it helps develop strength and control (although some students get so nervous about *adagio* that it makes them more tense). But we don't think *adagio* is anything to be nervous about.

Adagio also offers lots of room for creativity on the part of the ballet teacher. Some teachers give *port de bras* (*cambrés*), sometimes with one leg in *tendu* or *plié;* some devise stretches at the barre or *pirouettes* (though not for early beginners). Some give *fondus,* which are *pliés* on one leg. *Piqués* may be part of *adagio:* These call for the dancer to *plié* on one leg, then to extend and step out on the other leg, forward, side, or back. *Développé,* a favorite in the Joffrey School's adult classes, requires students to work on their extensions, control, turnout, and weight shift all at once. In short, there are simple *adagios* and more complicated combinations. Every *adagio* will be somewhat different. On the following pages, a primer for some *adagio* steps.

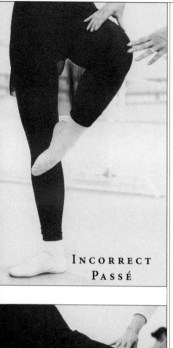

INCORRECT
PASSÉ

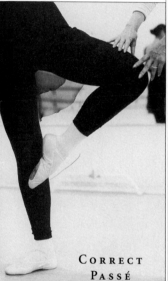

CORRECT
PASSÉ

Passé (or *retiré*): Technically the position is called *retiré*, and how you get there is called *passé*, but the two terms are frequently used interchangeably. Whatever your teacher calls them, they are among the most useful ballet steps and appear often in *adagio* and elsewhere. In *passé*, the working leg is bent, with the foot "attached" to the front, back, or occasionally the side of the knee of the standing leg. There are jumps with the leg in *passé*. And poses. And turns. In fact, it's the most common position for the leg in turns and any *passé* combination can be considered *pirouette* preparation.

The key to *passé* is always to keep the knee of the working leg turned out. When we teach *passés* to children, we tell them to "make a flag," and if you think of a flag waving at a 90-degree angle on a flagpole, you'll have an idea of what *passé* should look like. The foot is generally placed in the middle or slightly below the knee (although some teachers allow a somewhat lower *passé* if your turnout is weak). Beginners don't do *pirouettes* routinely (in most classes, they are just being introduced), but for those of you who are working on *pirouettes,* the best place for *passé* is as high as you can manage without lifting the hip.

Another trick with *passé* is to avoid sickling the foot. How to do that: If your *passé* is to the front, attach your little toe to the knee. If your *passé* is to the back, the inside of your heel is attached. *Passé* to the side is hardest to maintain without sickling your foot, but it's considered more advanced. In all directions, of course, remember to bring the inside of the heel forward.

Coupé: Coupés are the same as *passés,* only lower. Where the *passé* uses the knee as a point of orientation, the *coupé* uses the ankle. Keep your knee turned out, your heel forward, and watch for sickling here, too.

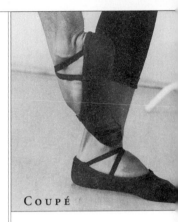

C O U P É

Fondu: It's not chocolate, or cheese, but there is a relationship between the meaning of the word *fondu* ("melted") and the movement. The best way to get a handle on *fondu* is to think of it as a *plié* on one leg, with both legs bending and both legs straightening at the same time.

Because the starting position of a *fondu* calls for the foot in *coupé,* you have to watch for sickling here, too. Another pointer: In *fondu,* the leg has a relationship with the audience, which means as you extend the leg you project your energy outward, not upward, and certainly not downward toward the floor.

F O N D U

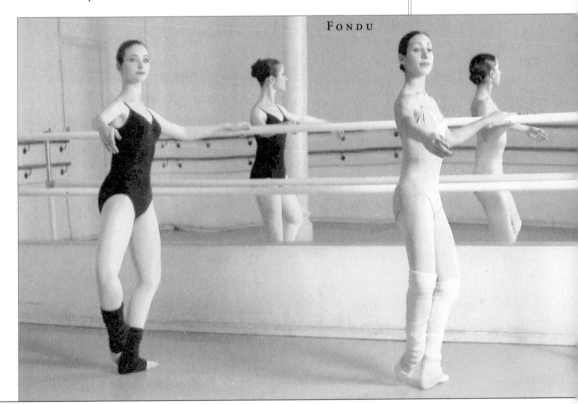

T H E   J O F F R E Y   B A L L E T   S C H O O L ' S   B A L L E T - F I T

Développé: Développé is one of the steps where it's easy to relate the word to the action. A *développé* starts in a *coupé* or a *passé,* then the leg opens or "develops" outward, to stretch and extend to its full length. Think of the *passé* or *coupé* as a bud, and the *développé* as the blossoming flower, and you have the idea.

In *développé,* although the height of the leg doesn't really matter, it's most impressive when it's high. The trick to achieving a high *développé* is to place the height of the *développé* with the knee, and not to drop the leg as you open it. As you unfold the leg, lift with the thigh, without distorting the line of the hip. And keep your turnout at all times. (Just keep in mind, at the beginning, form is more important than height. The height of your *développé* will gradually increase.)

Développé front is usually easiest to manage. *Développé* to the side can be tricky, because you're not really opening to the side at all. Unless you've got 180-degree turnout (rare at best), your leg will actually open to your second position (on a slight angle). When you *développé* back, your back should stay straight, but since your body has to give somewhere, bring your ribcage forward slightly, to balance the weight of the leg (don't bend from the waist). The look you're aiming for: as seen from the stage, a beautiful curve of the back that appears to be at a 90-degree angle to the extended leg.

Attitude: If you think of placing the foot in *passé* or *coupé,* and then lifting the working leg from the thigh, front, side, or back, you've got the "shape" of *attitude,* which is a lift of the bent leg. Then "wrap" the leg around yourself, keeping the knee and the toe at the same level. One of the tricks to *attitude,* and for everything else in ballet, is to open your thighs. You're not doing the Charleston. You can't do ballet with your thighs together.

Attitude *front* (devant) *is also called* tire bouchon (*corkscrew*) *because technically it's a different pose from* attitude *back. Anatomically, the leg can't create the same shape in the front as in the back.*

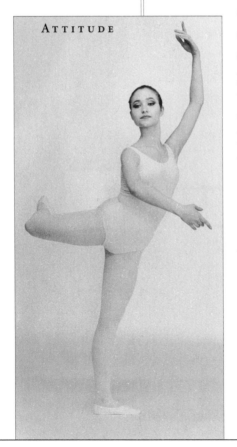

ATTITUDE

GRAND BATTEMENT

After *adagio,* the barre usually ends with *grand battements* in each direction; these are big, controlled kicks. Since they frequently come after *adagio* or another slower exercise like *rond de jambe en l'air* or stretches on the barre, they're quite brisk—your music will usually be a march—and they're fun.

To understand *grands battements,* think of them as growing out of everything else you've done at the barre—especially *tendu* and *battement tendu jeté. Grands battements* have the same brush against the floor, but they use more energy, and they're bigger—much bigger. That's where the *"grand"* comes in.

The key to *grand battement* is that it's not a lift but a push; it should use the inner muscles of the thigh, not the quads. Remember that the leg goes up briskly and is slow and controlled coming down.

Height, though nice, is not that important for the adult beginner; form is (as you gain strength in the back and buttocks, extension will come). And body alignment is an issue. When you do *grand battement* front, don't lean forward; stay straight. When you do *grand battement* back, the ribcage comes forward slightly. To the side, be sure that your weight is on your standing leg and that your working leg doesn't carry the whole body with it. In any direction, you are only moving from the hip socket and below. Your upper body should be perfectly still.

SOME DON'TS

Don't crease your leotard at your midsection (this means keep your back straight!).

Don't lift your leg with your quads.

Don't forget to begin your *grand battement* with your foot (it brushes along the floor).

Don't bend your knees.

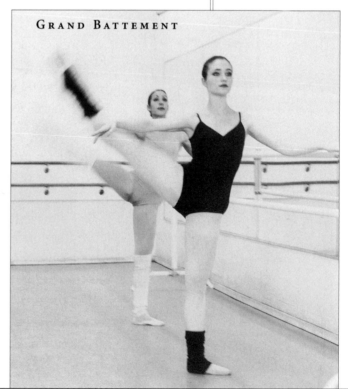

GRAND BATTEMENT

CENTER WORK

In a fitness book, the emphasis is naturally on the barre and floor exercises. But we like to think of center work as a reward. You've bought your shoes, you've been seen in public in a leotard, you've worked hard at the barre, and now you can dance! You don't want to? This is only a fitness activity? That's fine. But center is where it all comes together and a few stretches and jumps usually feel good after all that work at the barre.

In the Joffrey School's adult beginner classes, center work is progressive. At first, center is short—no more than a *développé* or *tendu* combination and some small jumps to finish up. As the class progresses, most students, even those coming in without much background, are able to do all but the *grand allegro* or big diagonal combinations. Small jump combinations (*changements, jetés, assemblés, sissones*) and *pirouette* preparations are choreographed

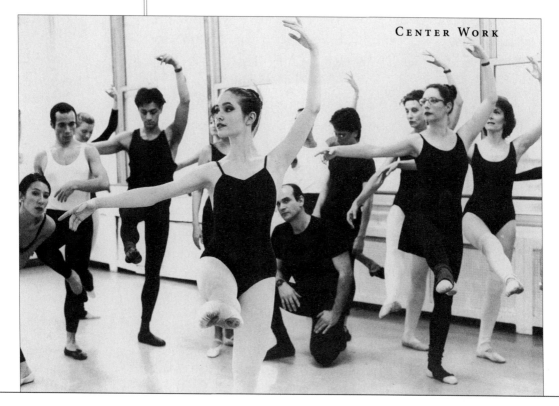

CENTER WORK

for the beginner and structured so that they serve as both intro-
ductory work for the absolute novice and practice for the more
experienced. If you're not inclined to participate, again, you don't
have to, but you can watch or "mark" the combinations until you
become comfortable enough to give it a try. Joffrey School adult
beginner classes are designed to get people comfortable enough to
try things they might not normally try.

Note: If you need extra attention, speak to the teacher about
walking you through some of the center combinations. Teachers
are there to teach and should be pleased when they're asked for a
little extra help.

Some Moving Steps

In your beginner ballet class you may be introduced to some moving steps. You'll probably see *glissade, pas de bourrée, piqué, chassé*,
and maybe even *chaîné* turns (which are not very popular, at least
according to one group of adult ballet students who contributed
questionnaires to this book). Below, a sampling of a few moving
steps that you will find in your adult beginner class.

♦ *Piqués* are an exercise at the barre, but in center are a way to trans-
fer weight from one leg to the other. In *piqué,* the standing leg
bends in *plié,* while the working leg stretches forward (or side or
back). During the *piqué* action, the body weight shifts all at once
from the standing leg to the working leg. As the foot reaches the
floor, you'll find yourself balanced in *relevé.* With this weight shift,
the standing leg ends up in *arabesque* or *attitude* or *passé,* and the
body weight is now over the leg that was extended. This actually
sounds far more complicated than it really is. In reality, *piqué* is a
quick and very natural motion (or at least as natural as ballet ever
is) and it takes far more time to explain it than to do it.

Piqué (which is an important step in beginner *pointe*) is one
reason adult beginners are encouraged to work hard on their *demi-*

pliés. If your *plié* is deep and elastic and the extended leg is very straight, the weight shift will take place easily and the resulting balance will be strong and steady. *Piqués* may be practiced at the barre before moving to center. Note: There is another related exercise, also called *piqué,* in which the foot of the stretched leg touches the floor briefly and is lifted (think of making "dots" on the floor). They're related because of the straight leg.

◆ *Pas de bourrée* is a neat way of changing feet, linking different steps together, and, like *piqués,* it is often practiced at the barre first. Some Joffrey School adult beginners told us that they find the *pas de bourrée* reminiscent of steps in folk dance or ethnic dance, which is a fairly good explanation. It's basically a step back, then a step side, closing in front (it can also be done in reverse). In the Joffrey School's adult classes, we often add *coupés* or *passés* to the step to make it more beautiful. When you do a *pas de bourrée,* try to keep the leg very strong and straight; remember, you're balancing on one leg, even as you change legs. And you never have both feet on the floor at the same time.

◆ *Balancé:* Teachers often add turns and choreographed arms to this step, but in essence, *balancé* is a classic waltz: It can be broken down into a big step to the side, followed by two little steps in place—but you know there's more to a waltz than that. With *balancé* comes a graceful, flowing motion (imagine yourself at a formal ball, in Vienna, before the turn of the last century). Keep the movement smooth and stretch the body. Your footwork should be "clean" (that means clearly defined, never fuzzy). Use your deepest *demi-plié* and your very strongest *relevé.* This is one place that the ballet fantasy will serve you in good stead.

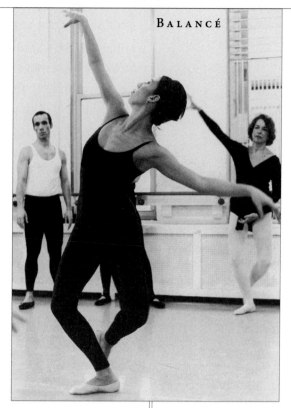

BALANCÉ

Center Turns (Learning to "Spot")

Pirouettes, piqué turns, and *soutenu* turns are all part of center (after they are practiced at the barre, that is). When you learn any of these and other turns, you will be expected to know how to "spot." Spotting is a ballet technique that keeps you from getting dizzy as you turn; it also gives the turn its characteristic ballet look. Unfortunately, spotting is seldom taught in adult beginner classes; it seems to be one of those things you're expected to pick up along the way. So here's how to go about it: When you spot you are simply whipping or snapping your head around as you turn (the body moves first, the head follows afterward). The first thing you do is choose something to look at. It could be the classroom clock, a picture on the wall, a taller student, anything at all. As you begin to turn, keep your eyes focused, then quickly snap your head around, so that you only lose sight of your spot for a fraction of a second. Think of the action when you shake your head "no," back and forth. The neck is relaxed and the shoulders stay down, allowing the head to move freely. Of course, you can do a turn without spotting, but chances are you'll get dizzy and thrown off balance. And, you'll never do more than a single turn.

Small Jumps

In center, the series of small jumps you will be learning are part of *petit allegro. Sautés* are small jumps in any position. There are *soubresauts* (jumps in fifth position), *changements* (jumps in fifth position in which you change feet), *pas de chat* (jumps with the legs in *passé*); *assemblés* (any jump from one leg to two), *sissones* (any jump from two legs to one), *jetés* (which are like *assemblés* except you land on one leg); and *échappés sautés* (jumps from fifth to second and back to fifth), to name just a few of the most common.

With all of these jumps, it's most important to begin—and end—in a springy and elastic *plié* (the *plié* you land in has to be the same *plié* you take off from for the next jump). A good *plié* is what gives your jump its spring and lightness and cushions its landing. Be sure you use your *plié*, however shallow it may be, and land with your heels down in the same elastic *plié*. Make sure you get high enough off the floor so you can point your feet. It is, after all, a jump.

Some jumps "travel," which simply means they move you across the floor, instead of staying in one place. This is just choreography; the how-to's are pretty much the same except for the weight shift which takes place in the air, so you can land farther away from where you started.

Diagonal Combinations

The diagonal combinations in center that end the class consist of traveling steps, which can make you feel like you're flying across the studio floor (they're really a lot of fun). In the beginner classes, we try to use vocabulary that we've worked on, for example, *balancé* or an *assemblé* that travels. Many teachers like to practice *grand jetés* or *grand jeté en tournant,* also called *grand jeté entrelacé.* Both require a strong *grand battement* to start with and a deep *demi-plié* to end with. The dancer should make sure she lands completely over her standing leg, in *demi-plié.* Be careful, though: These jumps have you landing on one leg, and an improper landing on one foot can be hard on the back and lead to injury. Watch your arms, too, which can sometimes cause the back to twist.

Note: One of the reasons that beginners of all ages, but especially adults, should not be given combinations beyond their level is that improper execution can lead to injury.

RÉVÉRENCE

Some teachers finish their class with what is known as a *révérence*—a curtsy or a bow (it's something you may remember from your childhood classes). It's a nice traditional way to end a class and shows mutual respect between the teachers and the students and acknowledges the pianist as well.

WHY HAVEN'T YOU COVERED . . .

What about *épaulement*? What about *batterie*? What about *fouettés* and partnering? *Ballotté, ballonné,* and *bourrée*? There's no question that we've left out a lot of vocabulary. Your class may be working on promenade or *assemblé en tournant*; and perhaps you have already done *pas de cheval* and *temps levé.*

We've tried to introduce, demystify, explain, and help build your ballet foundation. If you're ready to tell us what we haven't covered, then we've done our jobs. And you're probably ready to move ahead to the *Ballet-Fit* Workout that follows.

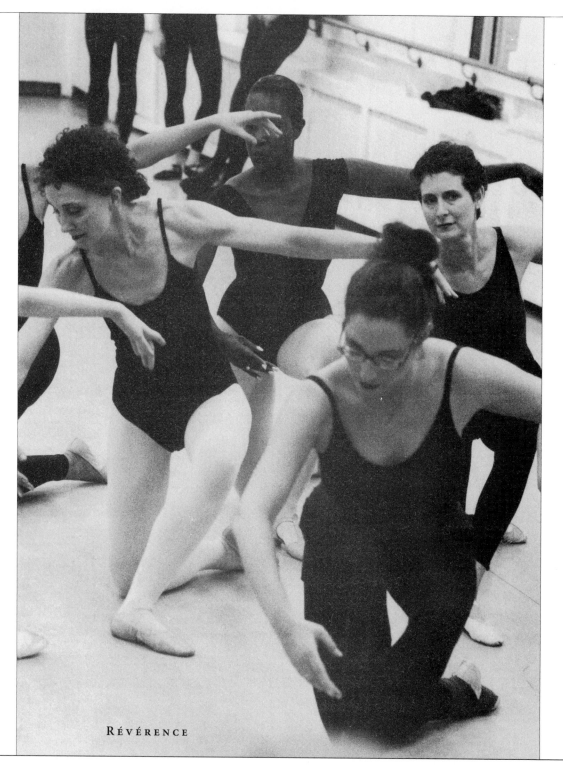

RÉVÉRENCE

Basic Barre and Center

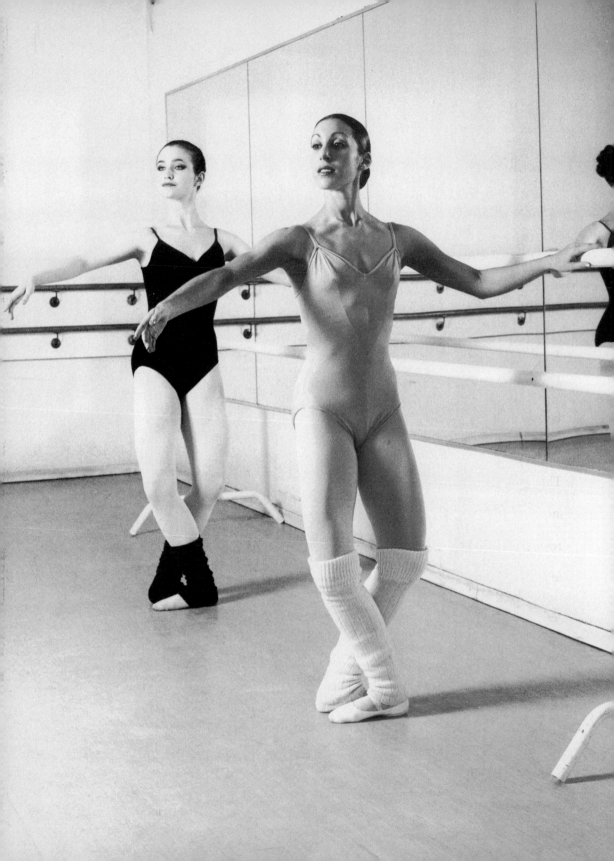

7

*P*utting It All Together: The *Ballet-Fit* Workout

❧

THE RESULTS-PRODUCING BARRE and floorwork in the 40-minute *Ballet-Fit* Workout here have been adapted from the adult classes given at the Joffrey Ballet School and can be done by anyone, anywhere, in the privacy of your own home or even in a hotel room when you travel.

The *Ballet-Fit* Workout emphasizes muscle toning, which means more definition and firmness to your muscles, and length, without developing excessive bulk. Your strength will improve, too (although keep in mind that the workout won't take the place of lifting weights if size and bulk are your goals). But again, performed two or three or more times a week, the *Ballet-Fit* Workout will help give an attractive shape and firmness to the muscles you have without adding bulk.

Before you get started, here are some tips to keep in mind:

♦ Before starting your *Ballet-Fit* Workout, *check with your doctor first,* as you would before beginning any exercise program.

- Work at your own pace. Ideally, if you are taking one outside ballet class a week, supplement it with two *Ballet-Fit* Workouts; if you are taking two ballet classes per week, one Ballet-Fit Workout may be enough.

- Set realistic goals. Some beginners are so enthusiastic about starting or being reintroduced to ballet that they try to do the workout every day. Not only is this too much to begin with physically, it will lead quickly to burnout, which means that in the long run you'll be less likely to stick with it.

- If you must have your ballet "fix" every day, do the stretches. They are safe to do everyday and will not only improve your flexibility and turnout and keep your movements fluid and more natural but will help promote circulation and make you feel more relaxed. You should always stretch—gently—*before* and *after* you exercise.

- Be creative with your time. You can do the *Ballet-Fit* Workout while you're watching the morning or evening news. Or in your office (close the door) during your lunch break. Create a weekly schedule that works for you by not holding yourself to the same workout time from day to day or week to week. For example, Tuesday at noon may work for you one week, but 4:00 may be better another week. Be flexible!

- As you progress, you can challenge yourself by doing the floor exercises with light (two- to three-pound) ankle weights or wrist weights that you can buy at a sporting goods store or by mail (start with one-pound weights and don't exceed four to five pounds). But avoid heavier weights, which can lead to injuries

---

BALLET-FIT WORKOUT FREQUENCY

Beginner: two times a week/hands on waist or shoulders.
Advanced Beginner: three times a week/add second position arms.
Intermediate: three to four times a week/add port de bras.

DECONSTRUCTING MORE BALLET-SPEAK

Ballet teachers use many exhortations so continuously that these phrases sometimes turn into ballet shorthand that newcomers don't fully understand. Keeping your back "straight," for example, doesn't mean military stance but refers to posture that's neither arched nor rounded (in other words, *in neutral alignment*). A "long" neck refers to the position of your chin. Don't thrust it out or tuck it under; it relates to the next command, "keep your shoulders down," which means being aware of the tension that can gather in the neck and shoulder region, causing the shoulders to contract and rise (it also means watching that you don't raise your shoulders when you raise your arms).

Keeping your hips "square" means facing forward, as much as you can. In real life, no one looks like an illustration. So we're asking you to be realistic about what your body can and can't do. In the case of movements to the back (such as *tendus* back or *frappés* or *grands battements*), it's difficult if not impossible for most people to keep their hips perfectly square—the human body isn't constructed to work that way, especially the adult body that hasn't been trained since childhood.

We've already explained pulling up (see page 90), but in brief, once again, it means trying to "lengthen" your body up and out of its hip sockets, engaging the abdominal muscles when you do. Keeping your heels "forward" means making sure you're using sufficient turnout when you point. To keep your arms from "drifting," check the mirror to be sure they're neither behind nor in front of your shoulder line. Review page 91 if you're sickling your foot. And try not to do it!

and promote bulky muscles—definitely not what we're after.

- Do every sequence slowly and with as much focus and control as possible. As a beginner, it's important for you to concentrate on doing each movement correctly, until your muscles remember on their own. As you master the *Ballet-Fit* Workout, consider using faster tempos, increasing the number of times you repeat the exercise, or changing them according to what your teacher is introducing.

- If you don't use music, keep counting in fours. Every ballet action is performed either on the count or the upbeat, so give each action its appropriate time. If it's a two-count *plié*, for example, bend your knees on count 1, and come up on count 2.

- As you progress, do the *Ballet-Fit* Workout near a mirror so you can watch yourself and self-correct. With or without a mirror, remember:

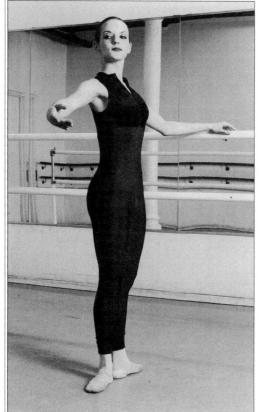

1. Keep your back straight.
2. Keep your neck long.
3. Keep your shoulders down.
4. Keep your hips square.
5. Pull up!
6. Keep your heels forward when you point your feet.
7. Stay aware of your arms (don't let them drift!).
8. Don't sickle your foot.

Before You Begin

Before you begin, find a workout "home." A kitchen counter or the back of a sturdy chair or stable piece of furniture is usually the right height (remember, your arm should never be higher than your shoulder, nor should your shoulder have to drop in order for your hand to rest gently on the barre). The available space should also be long enough and wide enough to allow your leg to extend fully, to the front, to the side, and to the back. And it should be unobstructed for your safety and that of your cherished possessions.

Whether a mirror is an absolute necessity depends on you. Often, ballet students, beginners to professionals, tend to become so involved with their reflected images that they forget to dance! Doing your barre without a mirror forces you to "feel" each movement; on the other hand, you may be "teaching" your muscles incorrectly. If you can use the mirror wisely, it will help you learn to correct yourself.

In addition, read each exercise all the way through before you begin, so you understand all the ballet movements called for. If you plan on using music, listen to it first and make sure the tempo (speed) is correct for you.

The Starting Position

Start your barre with your feet in second position (your toes face outward somewhat, your heels are aligned, and there is a space between your heels roughly equal to one of your own feet).

Pull your back up, your tummy up (*not* in!), and your shoulders down. You should not feel uncomfortable or unnatural, but you will look different: taller, thinner, and tighter. Place your left hand on your barre and your right hand on your waist or your shoulder, at first, then in second position, as you become more advanced. Breathe.

BEARING ARMS

As you become more comfortable with the barre, consider adding arms—*port de bras.* The arm traditionally goes to fifth *en haut* when the leg goes to the front; *à la seconde* (to the side, palm front) when the leg goes to the side; and *arabesque*, arm in front, palm down, at the same level as the shoulder, when the leg goes to the back. Remember to keep your shoulders relaxed, open, and *down*—in fifth position *en haut* or *arabesque*, especially. Unfortunately, it can be all too easy for beginners to lift their shoulders along with their arms.

Otherwise, keep your hand resting lightly on your shoulder—elbow up—or on your waist (a nice reminder to keep your posture erect) or *à la seconde* (which works the shoulders). If you choose *à la seconde*, be sure your arm doesn't drift backward, pulling your shoulder out of alignment.

Don't forget your preparation, either. Unless otherwise specified, start all exercises with arms *en bas*, then move your arm to first position (don't overcross in the front), then second position. Students tell us all the time that their arms are in better shape than ever, thanks to all of ballet's arm movements.

> The beauty of the *Ballet-Fit* Workout is that it's challenging but simple and not too high geared for a beginner to tackle. With the different modifications we've suggested, it's also as beneficial to bodies that haven't moved a muscle in months as it is to those who have been taking ballet all along.

The Ballet-Fit Warm-up

Some dancers make an effort to get to class early enough to warm up (although in theory at least, for dancers, *the class* is the warm-up for the day of rehearsals and performance).

For the adult, taking class is an end in itself, so we suggest the following series of preliminary stretches and bends to prepare the body to take maximum advantage of the ballet exercises to come. If it's at all possible to take any time to warm up, we recommend doing as many of the following as you can.

1. Start with basic shoulder raises (when we do these with children, we call them "hello shoulders, good-bye shoulders"). Simply raise your shoulders up and pull them down together, at least four times; then raise the right shoulder alone, then the left. Roll them backward and forward to loosen and relax your neck muscles; do this one four times in each direction.

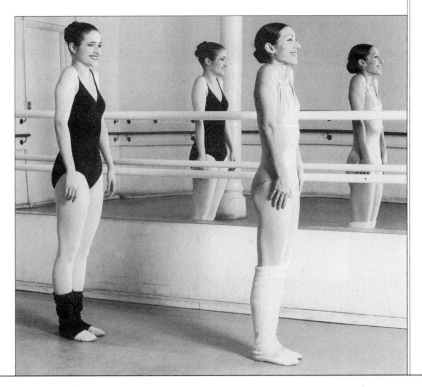

2. Next, facing the barre, with your feet parallel, do *tendus* to the front (as many as you have time for). You can also flex the foot or add circles of the ankle (*ronds de pied*) to warm up the ankle joint. Count to yourself in fours. All music and therefore all ballet is in multiples of four.

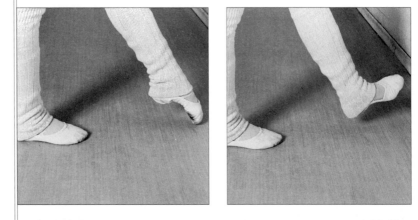

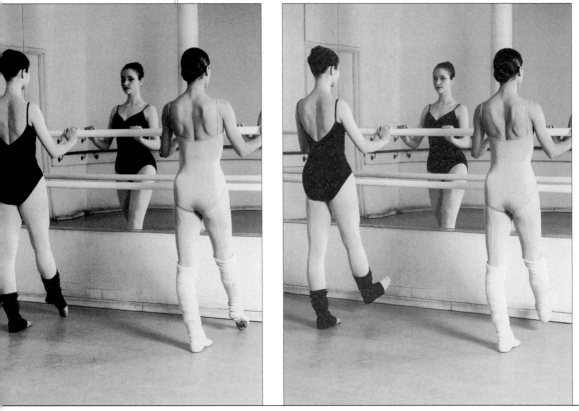

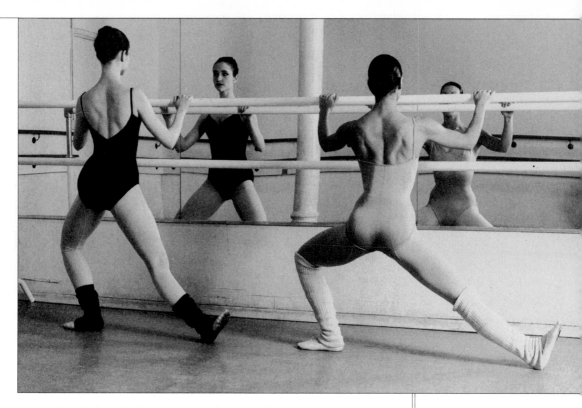

3. Again, facing the barre, do a few gentle *demi-pliés* in second position. You may want to *plié* on one leg while extending the other, foot flexed, then shift your weight so the other leg is bent (easy does it!).

Anyone can stretch. The important thing to remember is that we all differ in flexibility. When you carry out the stretches on these pages, we want you to stretch gradually, concentrating on the feel of the stretch, not how far you can go. Don't strain. Going too far can be painful and may leave you open to injury or with sore muscles for some time after.

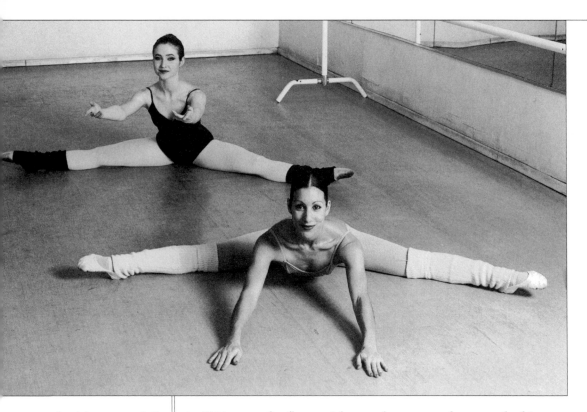

In doing some of the stretches, you may discover you have a "good" side and a "bad" side: One shoulder, knee, or leg may be stiffer than the other. Give the stiff side careful attention until it catches up with the good side. In this way, ballet can balance your body. At the same time, don't force any joint to bend or straighten if it doesn't want to. If your knee hasn't bent all the way in years, forcing it won't help.

4. Sitting on the floor, with your legs somewhat stretched in second position (not a split), reach forward from your hip socket, trying to reach your chest to the floor, and hold for at least 30 seconds. Come up, keeping your back flat at all times. Repeat. In the same position, now try stretching gently to either side, chest to knee. Just don't bounce or pulse. Although it may feel good, it will cause your muscles to tighten in reaction, the opposite of what you're trying to achieve! With any stretch, it's important to move slowly and deliberately and to hold the stretch for as long as possible. How long? Experts we've talked to vary in their opinions, but most advise between 30 and 90 seconds.

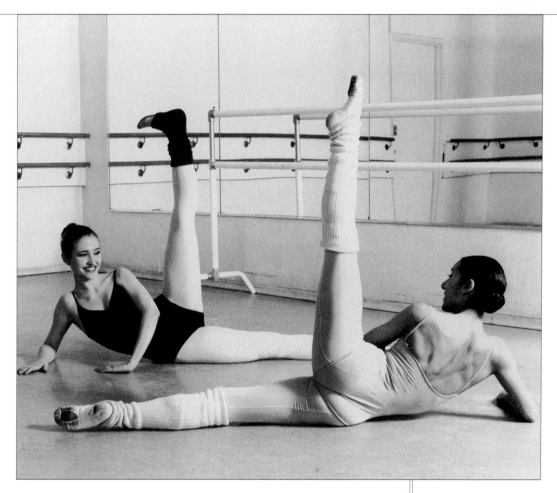

5. Lying on your side with your legs parallel, lift the top leg straight up and lower it smoothly. Aim for eight repetitions on each side, but try to do more as you master the warm-up; these are great for strengthening the outer hip (the abductors) and the inner thigh muscles.

To achieve turnout, the inner thigh muscles (the adductors) must be stretched also. To isolate and strengthen these muscles, do the above leg raises, but lift the *bottom leg* straight up, with the top leg forward, knee bent and out of the way.

Ballet requires a strong midsection to hold you up— abdominals are your "center": they support your spine and take your weight off your legs (especially important if you'd like to work *en pointe*, someday). This standard crunch works the upper abdominal muscles, and when you add a twist to it (as below), it works the obliques. In order to keep

6. Do some extra abdominal exercises that you don't usually do as part of your class, like crunches (see left "Crunch It!"). We hear that some dancers do hundreds every day, but we agree with personal trainers that eight to sixteen are enough to start with. Don't race through these, though; you won't get the most benefit. Crunches need to be done slowly and deliberately to get the most out of them. Be sure you do them with your lower back flat against the floor the entire time that you are lifting and lowering your upper body.

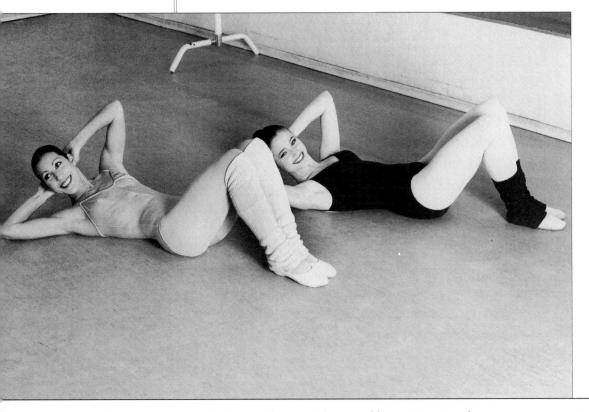

Putting It All Together: The Ballet Fit Workout

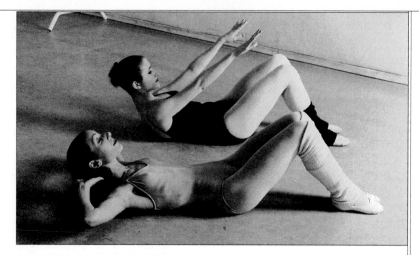

your head and neck aligned properly, conventional wisdom advises pretending you've got an orange or an apple tucked under your chin. Don't forget to support your head with your hands (or with a rolled-up towel), so you don't pull on your neck.

1. Lie on your back, arms clasped behind your head, knees bent, feet flat on the floor.

2. Consciously tightening the abdominal muscles and pressing your lower back on the floor, lift your upper body off the floor, with your chin level, your elbows at your sides. Hold; lower to starting position. Start with three sets of eight; work up to as many as you can. Exhale as you rise; inhale on the way down.

BALLET-FIT TIP

Use your abdominal muscles to power your lift by keeping your lower back firmly on the floor. Instead of clasping your arms behind your head, try resting your fingertips gently on your abdominals so you can feel them contract as you lift. If you're not used to abdominal work, don't forget to breathe, inhaling before your initial movement, exhaling on the lift. Some experts say that breathing brings oxygen to your muscles and helps alleviate next-day soreness to some degree. We find that stretching the next day also helps, but even so, we believe you should expect some degree of soreness, if not the next day then the day after. One way dancers like to "work through it" is with some *demi-pliés* in second position (and good old-fashioned aspirin). A warm bath may be good for the moment, but when you get out of the tub and your muscles cool and contract, you'll be sore again.

Soreness usually lasts about 24 to 48 hours (more than 48 hours means you overdid it). Your system does get used to the same warm-up exercises, though, so soreness should lessen in intensity and duration as you get used to the routine.

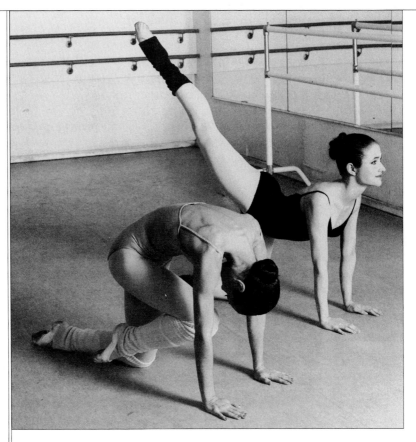

7. "Kitty Cats" seem to be among most exercise writers' favorites. Although we hear grumbling from students about them all the time, they are excellent practice for your *arabesques* and good for your gluteals besides. How to: In a kneeling position, start on all fours, with elbows straight and head level and eyes down. Then, bring your knee toward your nose and chest, bending your head to meet the knee, and in one continuous, graceful motion, lift your head up and *battement* your leg behind you. Your leg will reach the apex of the *battement* fully stretched, your foot will be pointed and your back will be arched. Bring your leg and head back to the starting position and repeat eight times with each leg. If your abdominals are weak, hold them in as you raise your leg. This will lessen the height of leg—and the amount of arch in your back—but it's much safer and just as productive.

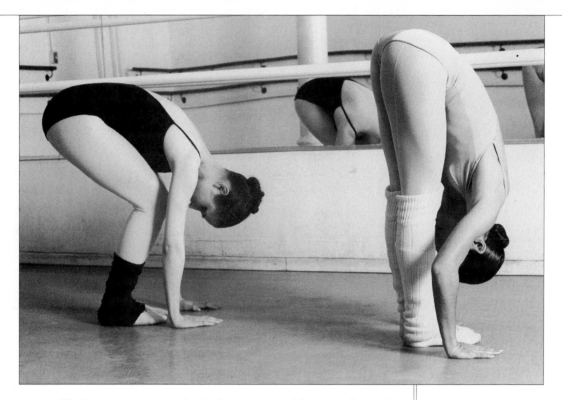

8. You'll also want to stretch the hamstrings (the muscles at the back of the thigh), which work together with the adductors to help achieve turnout.

Lie on your back, keeping both legs straight. Then lift one leg toward the ceiling. Clasp both hands behind your knee and gently pull your leg toward your chest, trying to keep the knee straight.

For a hamstring stretch, which also stretches the lower back (not for people with low back problems!), *demi-plié* with feet parallel, and bend forward from the waist, placing your palms on (or near) the floor; straighten the knees and hold that position for at least 30 seconds; then roll up.

BALLET-FIT TIP

Can't find 30 minutes for your *Ballet-Fit* Warm-up? Find 15.
Or 5. More is best, but some is always better than none, and
it's the consistency that counts.

9. To stretch the quadriceps (the big muscle that runs along the front of the thigh), stand straight, one hand on the barre for support if you need it, with the standing leg slightly bent (don't lock your knee). Bend the working leg, pulling the heel toward the buttocks with your hand. Hold for at least 30 seconds, then release. Repeat on the other side, two to three times for each leg.

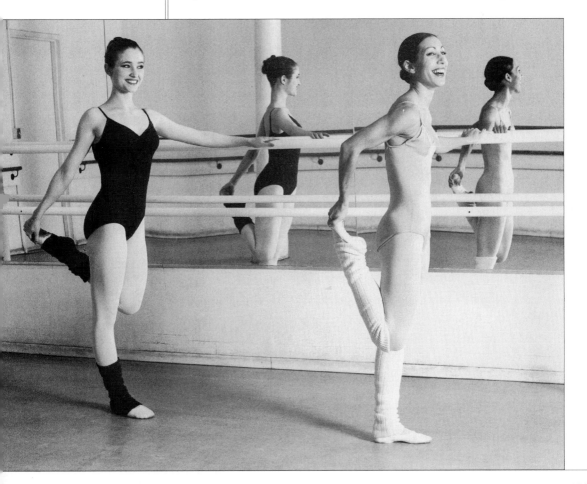

Putting It All Together: The Ballet-Fit Workout

Depending on the shape you're in, these last exercises may be too strenuous before your *Ballet-Fit* barre; you may not be ready for them. Use your judgment, but when in doubt, and if you're running short of time, put these off until after class and stick with the gentler stretches.

How much time should you spend warming up? It depends on how you feel and how much time you have. Some days you may only have 10 minutes, just enough to get in a few stretches, *pliés*, and some crunches. Other times, you may have a half hour and be able to do most of the warm-up exercises on this list. Feel free to select from these suggestions and do some but not others, or to substitute exercises according to your needs and preferences. You can also develop this warm-up into a supplementary workout for those days when you can't get to class, or time is too short for the complete *Ballet-Fit* barre. Just remember, be gentle. Again, don't bounce or pulse. It's counterproductive to the purpose of the warm-up. And do work up to more repetitions as you progress.

TAKE IT SLOW

Never rush through an exercise. If you do, you seldom work the muscles the exercise is meant to use. For example, as people do more sit-ups, they may use momentum, not muscle, to lift themselves, which also puts unnecessary strain on the back. While doing crunches or sit-ups, put your hands on your shoulders to avoid this, or to give yourself a more thorough workout (and take the heat off your back), curl up till your upper back is off the floor, then roll down at a slow, consistent speed.

The Ballet-Fit Workout

The *Ballet-Fit* barre that follows is an introduction to the basic ballet vocabulary and designed to create a structure to build on for at-home practice. As you become stronger and more advanced, we encourage you to add *relevés* and *port de bras*; if you wish, you can even change the combinations to make them longer or more complicated. We feel strongly, however, that for at-home adult practice, simple, straightforward combinations are best. When you don't have to worry about what comes next or where your arms go, you can spend more time and energy placing your body correctly, working the turnout from the hip, keeping the inside of the heel forward, and pulling the shoulders down. The results will show in class.

EXERCISE 1: DEMI-PLIÉS

DESCRIPTION: shallow knee bend.

COMBINATION: three *demi-pliés*, two counts each, in second, first, fourth, and fifth positions.

MUSIC: slow waltz, ¾ time (or count to yourself slowly, *one*, two, three; *two*, two, three, etc.).

HOW-TO: Starting with your left hand on the barre, feet in second position, right hand on the waist or shoulder, or *à la seconde*. Bend your knees sideways on the count of 1, straighten on 2, bend on 3, straighten on 4, bend on 5, straighten on 6, *tendu* on 7, close in first position on 8. Repeat in first, fourth, and fifth positions, finishing with feet in first. Then do *cambrés* (Exercise 2).

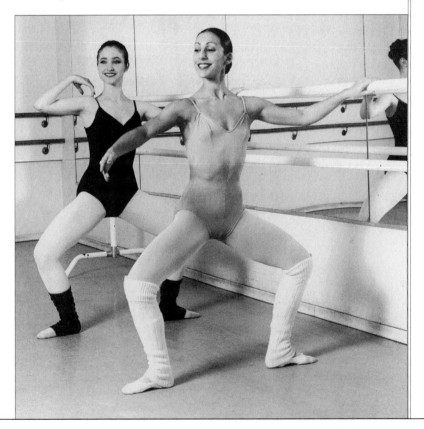

THE JOFFREY BALLET SCHOOL'S BALLET-FIT

OPTIONS FOR ADVANCED BEGINNERS: Do two *demi-pliés* and one *grand plié* (8 counts) and *cambré* forward and back (7 counts); *tendu* to first (on 8), and repeat in first position with *cambrés* to the barre and away from the barre. Repeat in fourth with *cambrés* forward and back. Repeat in fifth without *cambrés*. *Relevé* and balance, arms *en haut*.

BALLET-FIT TIPS

- The *plié* is an upward and outward action. You get "taller" and more pulled up as your knees bend. The heels stay down in all *demi-plié*.
- As you *plié* lift your hand slightly from the barre from time to time to test your balance in each position.
- After the third *demi-plié* in first position, point the right foot and slide it (*tendu*) in front of the left foot to fourth position (fourth and fifth positions are harder and you won't "go down" as far).
- In fourth and fifth positions, be sure to keep your hips as "square" as possible. Again, don't take being "square" too literally, though, or you won't be able to move!
- The slower and more deliberate your *pliés*—*demi-pliés* and *grands pliés*—the stronger your thigh muscles will become. This exercise also works the gluteals and the quads.

EXERCISE 2: *CAMBRÉS*

DESCRIPTION: bends of the upper body.

COMBINATION: *cambré* forward, back, and sideways to the barre and away from the barre, in first and fifth positions; 32 counts altogether.

MUSIC: same as *pliés*, ¾ time.

HOW-TO: You have finished your *pliés* with your feet in first position. Bend forward from the hip joint on count 1, keeping your back flat. When your back is parallel to the floor, on count 2, bend farther by rounding the back as if you were touching your nose to your knees and drop your head. Flatten your back and come up "in one piece" on counts 3 and 4. Turn your head to your right shoulder and bend back carefully on counts 5 and 6, keeping both shoulders even and using your upper back. Come

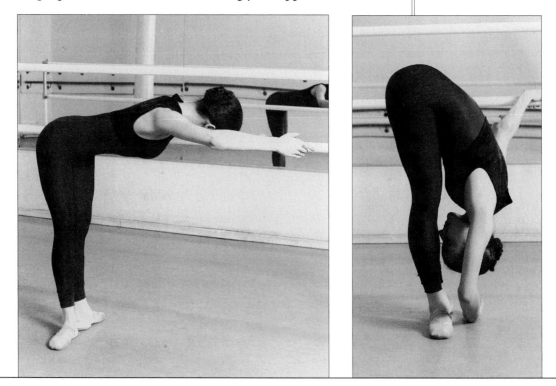

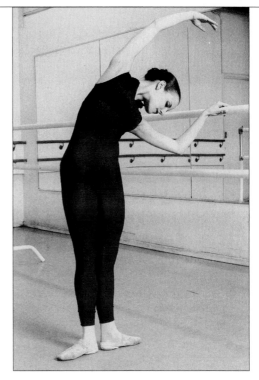

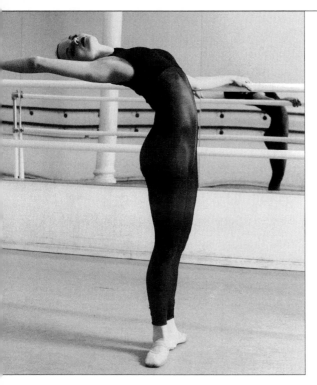

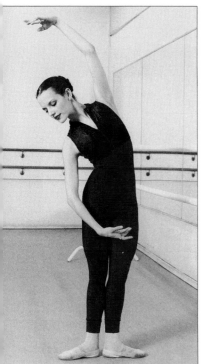

up on counts 7 and 8. Then reach toward the barre with your left shoulder by bending sideways and stretching your right side (counts 1 and 2), straighten up on counts 3 and 4, repeat the *cambré* away from the barre (counts 5 and 6), and straighten again (count 7). *Tendu* to fifth position on count 8. Repeat the *cambré* in fifth position, finishing with your right arm down and rounded.

> *Cambrés* are a good overall stretch to get you warmed up, open, and loose and also to work your back muscles. When you're doing *cambrés*, it's important to drop your head when you *cambré* forward (holding your head puts a strain on your neck, which we don't want).

Ballet-Fit Tips for *Cambré*

- Bend forward from the hip joint, not from the waist, by pulling your back up and taking a breath and "leading" with your chest. Think of reaching with the chest, not picking something up from the floor. (Note: If this movement causes you any back pain, bend only part of the way. If it persists, stop!)

- Even if you use your arms during your live class, when you work at home, you can keep your hand on your waist or shoulder to avoid pulling your shoulders up and losing the alignment of your upper body. Your body will learn how to control the shoulders this way.

- When you *cambré* to the side, again, don't reach with your arm, but stretch with your entire torso (keeping your hand on your waist or shoulder helps).

- Remember to turn your head to face your arm and bend backward only as far as you can go without sticking out your tummy or bending your knees, and keep your profile to the audience by looking at the inside of your elbow. You should feel a gentle stretch through the abdominals all the way down along the front of your leg. Always keep your legs straight and continue to pull up out of the hip socket.

- Try rolling up through the spine instead of keeping your back flat as you come up. This is a good way to release tension in the back and shoulders.

- When you *cambré* back, don't twist your body (think of your shoulders staying even with each other) and don't attempt a deep back bend. Compressing the lower vertebrae in your back can be dangerous if you have arthritis, disk problems, or chronic lower back pain. Instead, go with a natural arch to your own comfort level, and remember that everyone has different amounts of backward bend. If the position causes any pain in your spine, buttocks, or legs, try bending to only 50 percent of your full range of motion.

EXERCISE 3: *TENDUS*

DESCRIPTION: a systematic stretch of the leg and foot.

COMBINATION: *tendus en croix* (in the shape of a cross). Three *tendus* front; *demi-plié* and straighten up; three *tendus* side; *demi-plié* and straighten up; three *tendus* back; *demi-plié* and straighten up; three *tendus* side; *demi-plié* and straighten; *relevé* from your *demi-plié* and turn to the other side and repeat.

MUSIC: ¾ time or count 1,2, 1,2, not too fast.

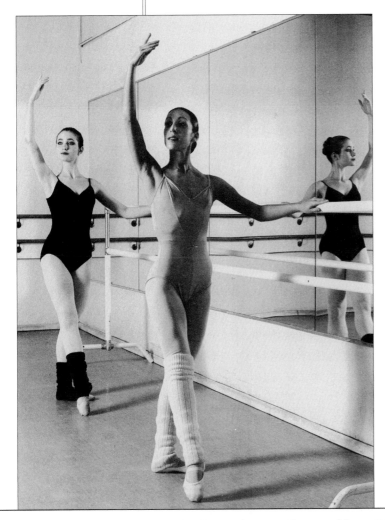

HOW-TO: Start with your feet in first position, left hand on the barre. Right hand may be at the waist, on the shoulder, or in second position. On count 1, push your right foot along the floor until gradually the foot is pointed, the leg is stretched, and only the very tips of the toes remain on the floor. On count 2, keeping the knee straight, pull your leg back to first position; repeat to the front, three times (counts 3, 4, 5, and 6) and *demi-plié* (counts 7 and 8); then side, then back, and then to the side again (32 counts in all).

BALLET-FIT TIPS

♦ Your foot should never leave the floor during the *tendu*.

♦ In each direction, make sure that the inside of the heel faces forward and your leg feels rotated. This is turnout!

♦ Be careful about directions. Front is in line with your nose; back is in line with your tailbone; side is a diagonal line from where your toes point in first position (not 180 degrees).

♦ When you *tendu* back, your working hip will "open," since anatomically it isn't possible to keep your hips completely "square" (facing front), but it is our ideal and a goal to aim for.

♦ Do not put any body weight over the working leg. The weight should be entirely over the standing leg.

♦ If you use a mirror, watch to see when you *tendu* to the back that the top of the foot is visible, not the profile. Tight hip flexors may prevent you from holding proper turnout when you *tendu* back, but do your best.

♦ To loosen tight hip flexors, try this: Kneel on the floor one foot forward, heel down, with the toes facing forward. Then tilt your pelvis so you lose the arch in your back and lean into the front leg until you feel a stretch in the front of the thigh of the back leg (see photograph, page 194).

OPTIONS FOR ADVANCED BEGINNERS

Do *tendus* from fifth position and add *port de bras* (arms *en haut, à la seconde, arabesque*). Remember to close alternately, in front or in back of your standing leg, when you do *tendus* to the side.

EXERCISE 4: OPTIONAL *TENDUS*

COMBINATION: *tendus en croix*, pushing the heel down to the floor each time, finishing in fifth back. *Passé* change, close front; *passé* change, close back; and repeat in reverse.

MUSIC: ¾ time (waltz time).

HOW-TO: Starting in fifth position, right foot front, left hand on the barre, right hand may be on the waist, shoulder, or in second position. Start the *tendu* on the "and" (the upbeat) and push the heel forward and down on count 1. You will now be standing on two feet with the weight equally distributed between them. Return to the *tendu*; that is, shift your weight back to the standing leg by pushing off with your working foot and close it in fifth position. Repeat to the side and to the back. *Passé* the working leg, closing front; and again, closing back. Repeat from back to front (16 counts in all).

BALLET-FIT TIPS

+ This is a weight-shift exercise! Be sure to start with your body weight entirely supported by your standing leg. When you push your heel down, you have shifted your weight from one leg to two legs.
+ As you push your heel down to the floor, articulate the foot. Go through the toes, the ball of the foot, and finally the heel. As you shift back to the supporting leg, use your toes and feel as if you're pushing the floor away.
+ Bring the heel forward as you push it down. Feel the muscles in the inner thigh. This works your turnout.
+ Use the foot the same way for the *passés*—"push off" with the toes. Keep the heel forward in *passé*—don't sickle!
+ Make sure your knee faces out in *passé*. Initiate the *passé* not only with the foot but with the thigh, using the thigh to lift the knee at the same time you push off with the foot.
+ Pay attention to your counts because we're using music differently here (we're starting before the count). The accent is on "heel down," or count it this way: *tendu* on "and," heel down on 1, *tendu* on "and," close on 2.

EXERCISE 5: *BATTEMENTS TENDUS JETÉS* (ALSO KNOWN AS *BATTEMENTS DÉGAGÉS* OR *BATTEMENTS GLISSÉS*)

DESCRIPTION: brushes with the foot.

COMBINATION: From first position, two *tendus*, two *jetés* in each direction, forward, side, back, and side (32 counts in all). *Demi-plié* to finish.

MUSIC: ¾ or ¼ (march time).

HOW-TO: Start in first position, left hand on the barre, right hand on your waist or shoulder or *à la seconde*. On count 1, stretch the foot forward in *tendu* front, then retract it to first position (2). Repeat (counts 3, 4). Then, to *jeté*, brush the foot

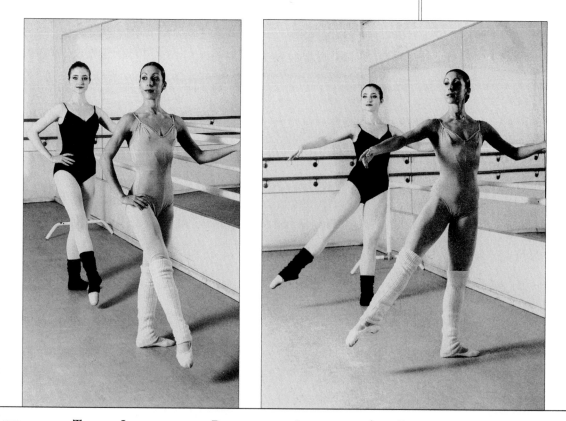

forward through *tendu* (5), lifting it off the floor a few inches, and back through *tendu*, closing in first position (6). Repeat (counts 7, 8). Then repeat from count 1, to the side, then to the back, to the side again. Finish in *demi-plié*.

BALLET-FIT TIPS
- The *jeté* springs off the floor with energy and an element of surprise.
- This combination is designed to illustrate the relationship between the *battement tendu* and *battement tendu jeté*. The action of a *battement tendu jeté* always includes a *battement tendu*. This means that the foot doesn't spring off the floor or return to its starting position until after the *tendu* is completed.

OPTIONS FOR ADVANCED BEGINNERS: Speed up your music. *Jetés* are fun to do at a brisk tempo and *very* strengthening for the entire leg. You can also work from fifth position, doing one *tendu* and two *battements tendus jetés* and a *demi-plié*, or eliminate the barre, keeping both arms *en bas* or *à la seconde*.

EXERCISE 6: RONDS DES JAMBES

DESCRIPTION: *tendu* in a semicircle.

COMBINATION: four *ronds des jambes en dehors, demi-plié* in fifth, outside foot finishes in the back. Repeat in reverse.

MUSIC: ¾ time.

HOW-TO: Start in fifth position, right foot front; left hand on the barre, right hand on shoulder, waist, or *à la seconde*. *Tendu* front on 1; move your foot to the side on 2, then back on 3, and close in first position on 4. Repeat *en dehors* a total of four times, finishing with *demi-plié* in fifth position, right foot back. Reverse, using the right leg. *Tendu* back on 1, to the side on 2, to the front on 3, close in first on 4. Finish in fifth with the right foot in front. Now do three *grands pliés* in fifth position (*demi-plié*, then go far-

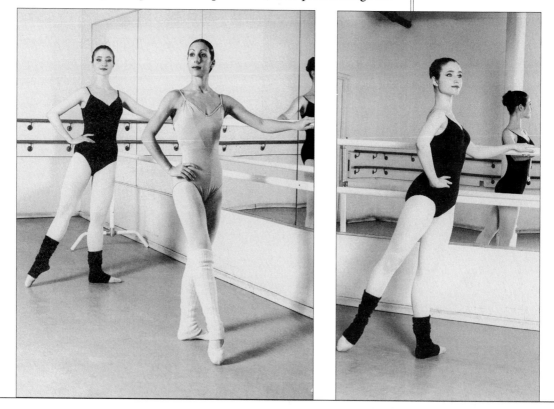

THE JOFFREY BALLET SCHOOL'S BALLET-FIT

ther so the heels lift from the floor, come up by forcing the heels down *before* the knees straighten). *Relevé* in fifth and turn to the other side. Option: If you wish to do your *ronds de jambe* again, finish with *cambrés* instead of *grands pliés*.

BALLET-FIT TIPS
- When you're doing *rond de jambe*, be conscious of the inside of the heel. Keeping the heel facing forward helps the leg rotate outward.
- It might seem harder to rotate the leg *en dedans*, so think of leading the leg with the inside of your heel.
- Going "through" first position should remind you to keep your turnout. As you do, be careful not to bend your knee.
- Always go "through" the *demi-plié* on the way to the *grand plié*, and as you come up.

OPTIONS FOR ADVANCED BEGINNERS: Speed it up. Use ¾ time (march time) instead of a waltz. Start with a preparation: *plié tendu* front, then straighten the standing leg as you open to the side.

EXERCISE 7: *FRAPPÉS*

DESCRIPTION: brushes of the foot from *coupé* (bent knee).

COMBINATION: four *frappés* forward; four to the side; four back; four side; finish in first position. Repeat on the other side.

MUSIC: ¾ time.

HOW-TO: Start in first position, left hand on the barre,
right hand on the waist or *en
bas*. Prepare on counts 1 and 2,
keeping the right hand on the
waist; on count 3 *tendu à la seconde*; on count 4, place the
flexed right foot in *coupé* with
the heel resting above the ankle
of the standing leg. From the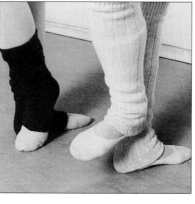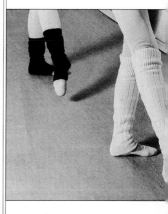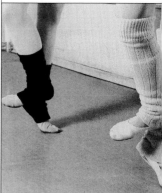
coupé position, brush front, pointing the foot on count 1; retract
it on count 2, and repeat three more times for a total of 8 counts.
Repeat to the side, to the back, and to the side again, and finish
in first. Turn to the other side and repeat with the left foot.

BALLET-FIT TIPS

- Remember that *frappé* is a sharp, sprightly action, not slow
  or lyrical.
- When you retract the foot, be sure to return to the correct,
  flexed *coupé* position (one Joffrey adult remembers the
  placement of *coupé* by positioning her foot exactly where
  her footless tights end).
- *Frappé* to the side can be tricky because the placement of
  the *coupé* differs from front to back. In *coupé* front, the outside of the heel rests on the standing leg, but in *coupé* back
  the inside of the heel rests on the standing leg. When we do

frappé à la seconde, the *coupé* alternates between front and back. Note: You might remember the "wrapped foot" from your childhood training. We prefer the foot-strengthening effect of going from the flex to the point.

- The *frappé* can be hard to learn (and alternating front and back makes it more complicated). Choose slower music and be patient with yourself.

OPTIONS FOR ADVANCED BEGINNERS: Keep the foot pointed and touch the floor in *piqué* (or *pointe tendu*) and don't brush against the floor. Think instead of projecting outward with a beautiful, stretched foot. Do the entire combination *en relevé* with a pointed foot. Practice double *frappés,* if and only if you have had them in class (*coupé* back, *coupé* front, brush foot front; *coupé* front, *coupé* back, brush side; *coupé* front, *coupé* back, brush back; *coupé* back, *coupé* front, brush side).

EXERCISE 8: ADAGIO

DESCRIPTION: slow, stretched, controlled movements.

COMBINATION: *passé, développé, piqué* (*pointe tendu*), close in fifth position, to the front, the side, and the back, finishing with the right foot in back. *Fondu*, open side; close front and turn to the other side. Arms may remain in second or *en haut* or *arabesque*, as below.

MUSIC: ¾ (slow).

HOW-TO: Start in fifth position, left hand on the barre, right arm in second. On count 1, with arm in first (picture 1) lift the outside leg to *passé*, stretching it (*développé*) in front on count 2, lifting the thigh and opening from the knee to "develop" the full, extended leg and moving the arm *en haut* (picture 2). Put your leg down gently on the floor and *piqué* (*pointe tendu*) on count 3, and close, as you would in *tendu*, on count 4, in fifth front.

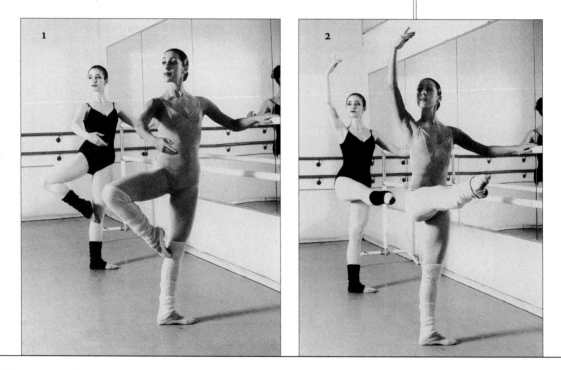

THE JOFFREY BALLET SCHOOL'S BALLET-FIT

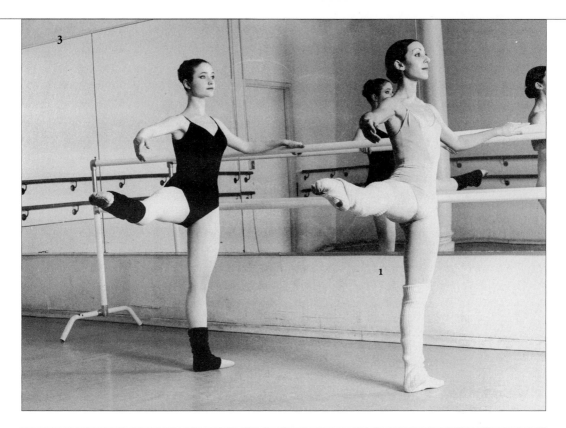

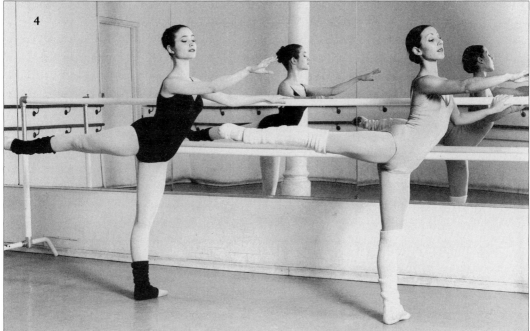

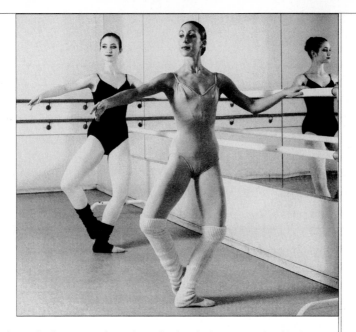

Repeat to the side (picture 3) and to the back (picture 4), closing in back each time. Then *fondu* by bending both legs on 5, extend the outside leg to the side, straightening the standing leg at the same time on count 6. Bring the legs tightly together on 7 and turn to the other side on 8.

BALLET-FIT TIPS

- Don't forget to move the arms with the legs, or leave the arms in second position throughout.
- Be sure to keep your knee facing outward (not forward) in *passé*.
- Keep the turnout as you *développé* the leg (open the leg from *passé*, but don't let it drop).
- We don't emphasize how high you lift your leg in *développé*, but you should keep it at least 45 degrees, if not 90 degrees. The way to do this is by lifting from the inner thigh as you begin to open and extend the leg. Keep your foot stretched and "reaching" so it stays pointed and turned out.
- In the *fondu*, both legs bend and straighten at the same time.

EXERCISE 9: GRANDS BATTEMENTS

DESCRIPTION: big kicks.

COMBINATION: three *grands battements* in each direction, with a *demi-plié* in between. Turn and repeat on the other side.

MUSIC: ¼ (big march).

HOW-TO: Start with your hand on the barre, right arm on waist, shoulder, or *à la seconde*. Feet in fifth position, right foot front. Prepare in four counts, holding the arm in second position (or, if you choose, with the *port de bras* described in the Options for Advanced Beginners, following). Push the foot hard against the floor so the leg swings up on count 1; place it carefully in *pointe tendu* front on the "and" (upbeat); close in fifth position on count 2. Repeat three times and *demi-plié* in each direction for a total of 32 counts.

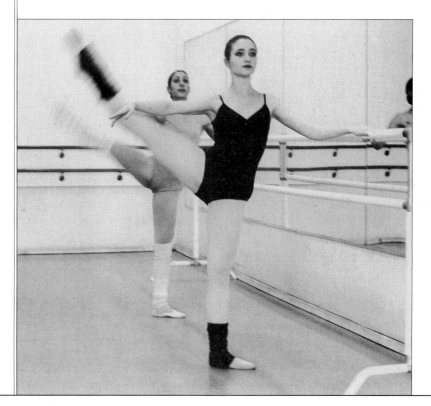

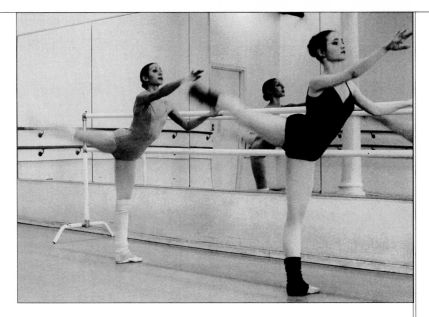

OPTIONS FOR ADVANCED BEGINNERS: Try doing the *grands battements* without holding the barre, using the abdominals for control. Or add *port de bras*: arms *en haut* when your leg goes front, *à la seconde*, when your leg goes to the side, and *arabesque* arm, when your leg goes to the back.

BALLET-FIT TIPS

- *Grands battements* should be done with energy (for music, think military march!). The back stays long and the leg is pushed up rather than lifted.
- The action is fast and energetic on the way up, slow and controlled on the way down, going "through" the *tendu* as in the *battement tendu jeté*. Try not to let your body move back and forth as your leg moves up and down.
- In second position, stay strong, firm, and pulled up and make sure your weight remains over your standing leg.
- Lean forward slightly from the ribcage when doing *grands battements* to the back. Keep your leg directly in line with the heel of your supporting foot (don't let it swing to the side).

FloorPlay

Ballet-oriented floor exercises have become something of a signature of the Joffrey Ballet School's classes to help adult beginners gain strength and flexibility as quickly as possible. Without strength (which can be developed) and flexibility (which can be increased) there is no dance. Just keep in mind that it's hardly necessary to be able to do a split; in fact, for some people, it may even be dangerous. Adults don't heal as well or as quickly as children do, so exercise, but exercise caution, as well.

The exercises that follow take place on the floor, a safer option than stretching on the barre because the floor provides a stable surface with a good base of support for your entire body. Hamstrings and adductors (the inner thigh muscles) are especially vulnerable on the barre, and knees have a tendency to be pushed into hyperextension (which means bent backward). Plus, it's harder to relax while you're trying to balance on one leg!

FloorPlay/Exercise 1:
Second Position Stretches

BODY BENEFITS: stretches the hamstrings, the inner thigh muscles (adductors), and the lower back, and lifts the body up out of the hip socket.

1. Sit on the floor, back straight, legs open to the sides in a V. Don't force your legs open wider than is comfortable, and make sure your legs rotate outward from the hip. Don't let your legs roll inward. A good way to check is to keep your knees facing up.

2. Pull up out of your hip socket, freeing the upper body to work "in one piece." Your arms may be in fifth *en haut*, or your hands may be on your shoulders to help keep them down.

3. Now bend to the right from the hip socket, reaching to the side, trying to place your right ear on your right knee. Don't force and gently hold this stretch for seven slow and steady counts. Don't bounce or pulse.

INCREASING TURNOUT

What's nice about this stretch is that it does great things for your turnout. You'll not only use what you have, you'll increase it, too. It also helps to lengthen some of the muscles (although not all) that you need for turnout. Keep in mind, though, that muscles are like elastic bands. Even though you stretch them, they spring back to their

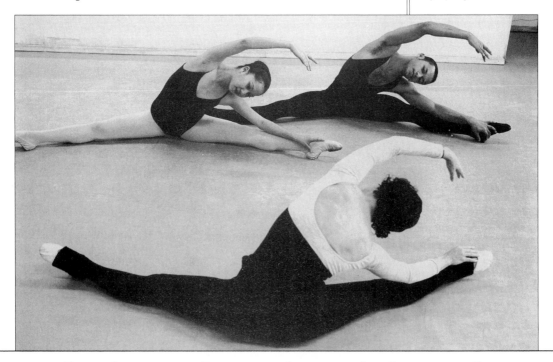

THE JOFFREY BALLET SCHOOL'S BALLET-FIT

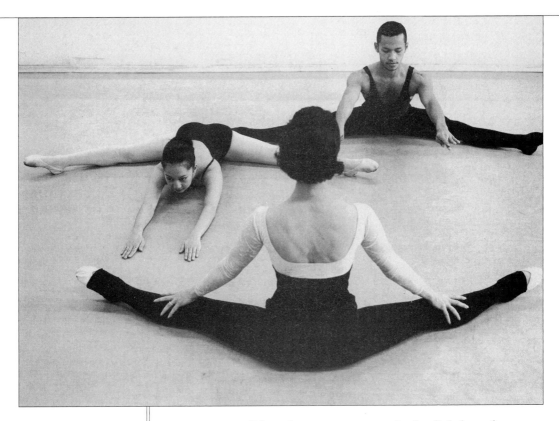

original length quickly. That's why dancers are always stretching! But although it takes many, many stretch sessions, patience and a good warm-up can make a difference in muscle length and flexibility, which can increase over time.

4. On count 8, lift and turn your upper body slightly to face your right leg. Then stretch for an additional seven counts. Come up on count 8.

5. Repeat to the left side.

6. Pull up and stretch forward, maintaining the rotation of your hips. Lead with your chest and stretch gently for two sets of eight counts. Your goal is to put your chest on the floor, but it doesn't matter how far you actually go as long as you keep your back flat (not rounded or arched) and your legs stretched and rotated. Come up on the sixteenth count.

7. Reach to your right on count 1, to the front on count 2, left on 3, and up on 4, making a circle with your upper body. Reverse, going from left to right in four counts, and repeat again, to the right, to the front, and to the left, for a total of 16 counts.

FLOORPLAY/EXERCISE 2: DOUBLE LEG LIFTS

BODY BENEFITS: strengthens the lower abdominal muscles.

1. Lie on the floor, spine flat (think of pressing your navel into the floor). Extend the legs in front of you. You may do this with your feet turned out or parallel. Keep your arms on the floor in second position.

2. Slowly raise both legs to a 45-degree angle (count 1) and slowly lower them until they are just a few inches off the floor (count 2), feeling your abdominals contracting as you lower. Start with 16 counts and build up to 64. In order to do this exercise correctly, your lower back must be pressed tightly to the floor.

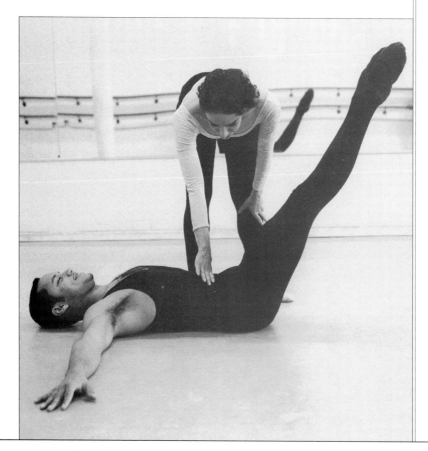

- If you have weak abdominal muscles to begin with, the exercise above is not right for you. It would require you to rely on your hip flexors for the lift, which will stress your back, hyperextending the lumbar spine. To improve weak abdominals, try doing these leg lifts one leg at a time, alternating from the right leg to left.

- If one-leg-at-a-time leg lifts continue to strain your back and cause your pelvis to rotate, don't be proud. Pass them up and substitute an easier variation that also works the lower abdominals: Lie flat on your back, knees bent, feet on the floor, arms at your sides. Then bring your right knee, in the bent position, to your chest on count 1, extend your leg (turned out and foot pointed) on count 2; then lower it down to the floor on 3. Alternating legs, do 16 lifts to start, build up to 64 as you gain strength. Just remember, it's form that is important here, so it's quality, not quantity, we're after. Keep your back pressed to the floor and your abdominals *tight*!

BODY BENEFITS: works the abdominals, stretches the hamstrings and adductors.

1. Sit up, back straight, legs stretched in front of you (turned out, feet pointed), arms *en haut* (shoulders down).

2. Reach forward with the chest, keeping your arms rounded (try to put your nose on your knees) on count 1. Using your abdominals, return to sitting position on 2, *slowly* roll down to the floor, one vertebrae at a time, through the spine, tailbone first on 3 (use the abs to control the movement). Return to starting position, arms *en haut* on 4. Start with 8 sit-ups (32 counts), and work up to 24 (96 counts). Note: Be sure to roll down *slowly* on count 3. If you come down too quickly, you won't recruit your abdominals (most of your momentum will come from your arms and trunk), which defeats the purpose of this exercise.

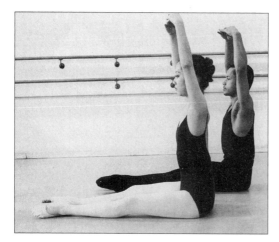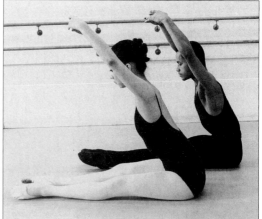

BALLET-FIT POINTERS AND MODIFICATIONS
- If you have very strong abdominals, on your third set of eight, open your legs to second position on the first count, then close them on the second (but don't do this until the original movement is easy!).

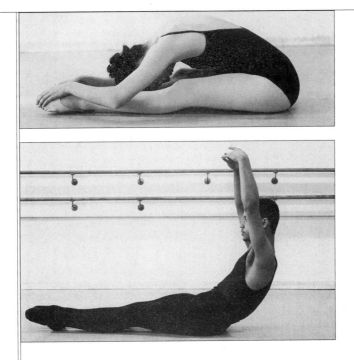

- ◆ If you tend to use your arms for momentum or if you find you rely on your back muscles, not your abdominals, try doing this sit-up with your hands resting on your shoulders. You can also slow down the count so it takes twice as long to do the same number of repetitions.

- ◆ You can substitute partial sit-ups, done with bent knees, as follows: Lie on the floor, knees bent, feet flat on the floor, arms behind your head on the upper neck (fingers touching), and elbows out to the side. Contract your abdominal muscles, bringing the lower part of your pelvis toward your head, causing your back to press flat into the floor (this is known as a pelvic tilt). At the same time, lift your head, neck, shoulder blades, and upper chest off the floor, toward the ceiling. Be sure to keep your back flat, your elbows out to the sides, and support your head with your fingers (don't pull it with your hands). Hold for five seconds and lower slowly half way down. Lift and lower eight times; work up to three sets of eight.

FloorPlay/Exercise 4:
Rond de jambe en l'air

BODY BENEFITS: opens the hip joint and increases rotation; strengthens the abdominals and adductors.

Lie on the floor, arms at your sides or with your hands resting lightly on your hips to see that they move as little as possible (when your hips are still your abdominals are working).

1. Slowly raise your right leg into *passé* (1) turned out. *Développé* in front on 2, then lift and rotate *à la seconde* on 3, and close on 4. Repeat with the opposite leg. This is an *en dehors* action.

2. Next, slowly *passé* your right leg on 1, *développé à la seconde* on 2, rotate to the front on 3, close on 4. Repeat with the other leg. This is *en dedans* action.

3. Do the complete exercise, *en dehors* and *en dedans*, four times (64 counts).

BALLET-FIT POINTERS AND MODIFICATIONS

♦ This is an adaptation of more advanced ballet vocabulary. If you are doing *rond de jambe en l'air* at the barre or in center, you would be on your standing leg for a long time. On the floor you get the benefit of the exercise without the need to balance on one leg.

♦ Pay attention to keeping your torso stable and flat against the floor. Don't twist your hips or shoulders.

♦ If you do it right, *rond de jambe en l'air* works the abdominals as well as the turnout.

♦ Modifications: None really. As long as the movement is slow, controlled, and deliberate, this exercise is good for everyone.

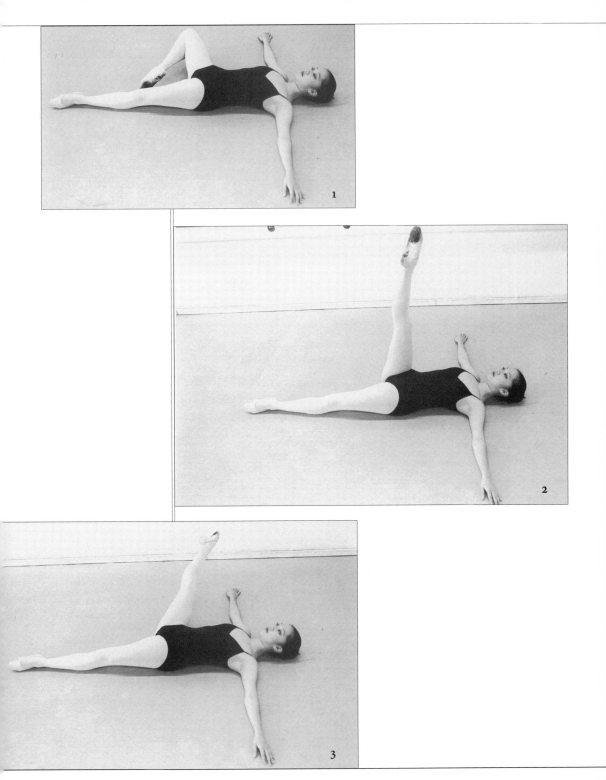

FLOORPLAY/EXERCISE 5:
ENTRECHAT SIXES

BODY BENEFITS: strengthens the upper and lower abdominals and the inner thigh.

1. On the floor, lean back, elbows and forearms propping up your upper torso (this is a good position for the lower back because the abdominals can be easily recruited and the pelvis supported). Extend your legs, turning out from the hip socket. Lift your legs anywhere between 45 and 90 degrees (your own comfort level) with the right foot on top of the left (fifth position). The higher you lift, the easier this exercise becomes. Start with your legs higher, then, as you get stronger, lower your legs without arching your back off the floor, using your abdominals, not your hip flexors or back.

2. With your legs extended and lifted, open legs to the side and cross your left foot in front of your right, then cross them again and hold. Repeat (the count is one, two, three, hold four). Do 16 counts, then stop. If you can do these comfortably, then lower your legs a little and do 16 more counts, working up to 64 or more.

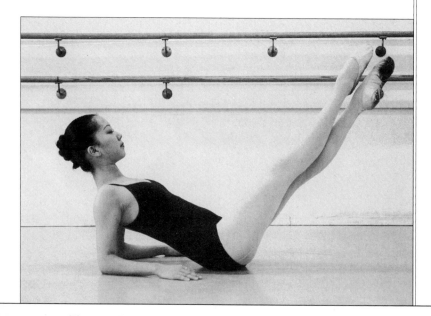

THE JOFFREY BALLET SCHOOL'S BALLET-FIT

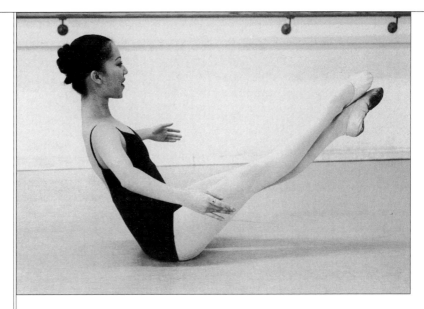

BALLET-FIT POINTERS AND MODIFICATIONS

- You have to have very strong abdominals to do *entrechat sixes*, which are preparation for a group of advanced jumps called *batterie* in which the legs make a scissorlike movement in the course of the jump. The key to doing this exercise correctly is to avoid using your hip flexors. When the abdominals aren't strong enough, most people fall back on their hip flexors, which is not what we're looking for. Think in terms of really working the abdominals and do as few as you need to feel them working.

- The strengthening benefits of *entrechat sixes* are dependent on consistency. If you can do these every day, you will see a dramatic improvement in your abdominals. But you have to do them every day!

- What if you're really strong? Try this variation as a challenge: Take your arms off the floor and do your *entrechat sixes* with your body balanced in a shallow V and your weight on your tailbone. Brava!

FloorPlay/Exercise 6:
Push-ups (Men Only)

BODY BENEFITS: strengthens the chest, shoulders, and upper arms.

Classic Push-up

1. Stretch out on the floor in the standard push-up position: facing the floor, supported by your hands and toes (don't lock your elbows).

2. Lower your body slowly to the floor by bending your arms; when you reach the floor, straighten arms to raise up. Do not arch your back. Instead, keep your back flat and your buttocks low and squeezed tight. Keep a conscious tightness in your abdominals, too, so that they can contract isometrically.

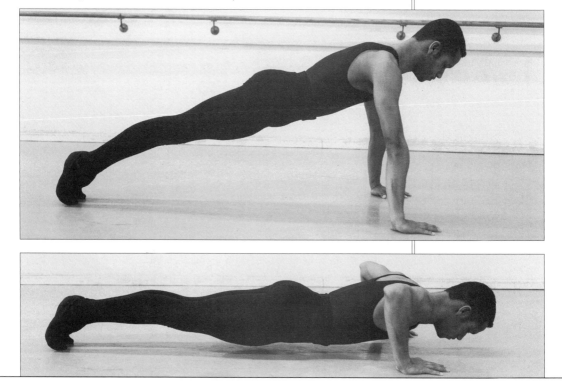

THE JOFFREY BALLET SCHOOL'S BALLET-FIT

Hip flexors are the muscles that go through the pelvis, connecting your thigh bones to your lower spine. Since they are major muscle movers as well as stabilizers, they are used when you swing your leg forward or when you kick or lift your leg up. When you're standing *en relevé*—on *demi-pointe*—it's the hip flexors that stabilize your trunk. Try not to use them, though, when you lift your leg in movements like *grand battement*; they get enough use (and when you do use them the abdominals shut off). Instead, when lifting your leg in class, let your inner thigh muscles share the load with the hip flexors. Of course, if you're not using your turnout, you'll wind up using your poor, overworked hip flexors again. Plus, when you're standing, if you're not activating your abdominals and gluteals enough to stabilize your trunk, your hip flexors tend to kick in again, to help.

MODIFICATION PUSH-UP FOR WOMEN (OPTIONAL)

1. Start on your hands and knees, with your palms flat and slightly more than shoulder distance apart. Keep your hands immediately under your shoulders.

2. Keep your back straight, raise your lower legs off the floor and cross your feet at the ankles. To avoid putting too much pressure on the knees, place your weight slightly above the kneecap, where there's a bit more padding.

3. Lower your torso and head slowly, until your elbows are parallel to the floor and repeat. Be sure not to lock your elbows on the "up" position. A reminder: For both men's and women's push-ups, inhale on the way down and exhale on the way up.

FLOORPLAY/EXERCISE 7: THE HIP FLEXOR STRETCH

BODY BENEFITS: stretches the hip flexors.

Kneel on the floor, one knee bent with the foot flat on the floor in front of you, back straight, arms at your sides. Push forward on the front leg, feeling the stretch in hip flexor of the back leg. Hold for 30 seconds, repeat three times; then change legs and repeat.

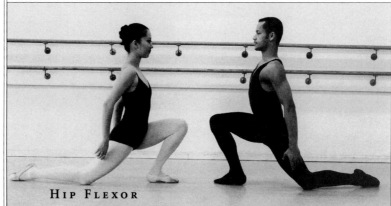

HIP FLEXOR

FLOORPLAY/EXERCISE 8:
THE BUTTOCKS STRETCH

BODY BENEFITS: stretches the back, the hamstrings, and the gluteus maximus—and it feels good.

Sit on the floor, back straight, crossing your legs loosely (don't pull them close to the body). Then, lifting your buttocks off the floor, reach forward with your chest, keeping your back as flat as possible. "Walk" on your hands, forward to the right, then to the left, exaggerating the stretch by pulling forward with your hands. Hold for 20 to 30 seconds; then change legs.

These floor exercises are wonderful to do at home, before your class, or while you are traveling. And regardless of your current fitness level, or how many ballet classes you are taking, you'll get results faster if you integrate this workout into your regular fitness plan and, most important, if you do it consistently. Keep in

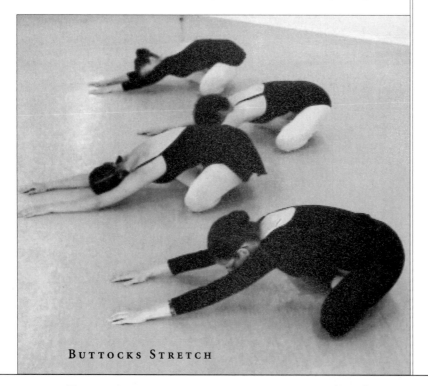

BUTTOCKS STRETCH

mind that maintaining a healthy and *Ballet-Fit* body is an ongoing process that calls for patience, persistence, and perspiration.

Ballet-Fit Pointers and Modifications

- If you're a beginner and not very flexible, modify this stretch by bending one knee so you can concentrate on stretching one leg at a time. (Remember that bodies are often asymmetrical; one leg may be more flexible—have more "stretch"—than the other.)
- You can also make a smaller V during the stretch, and eliminate the forward stretch, stretching only from side to side.
- If your back hurts while doing this exercise, you may not be doing it correctly. Be sure to keep your back straight and flat and to lift up out of the hip socket. If you have a bad back, it is always best to stretch only to the point of comfort. If getting up from a prolonged stretch is painful, spend less time in the forward bent posture. If it is still painful, lie on the floor and pull or bring your legs (straight or bent) into your chest while keeping your head and neck in contact with the floor.

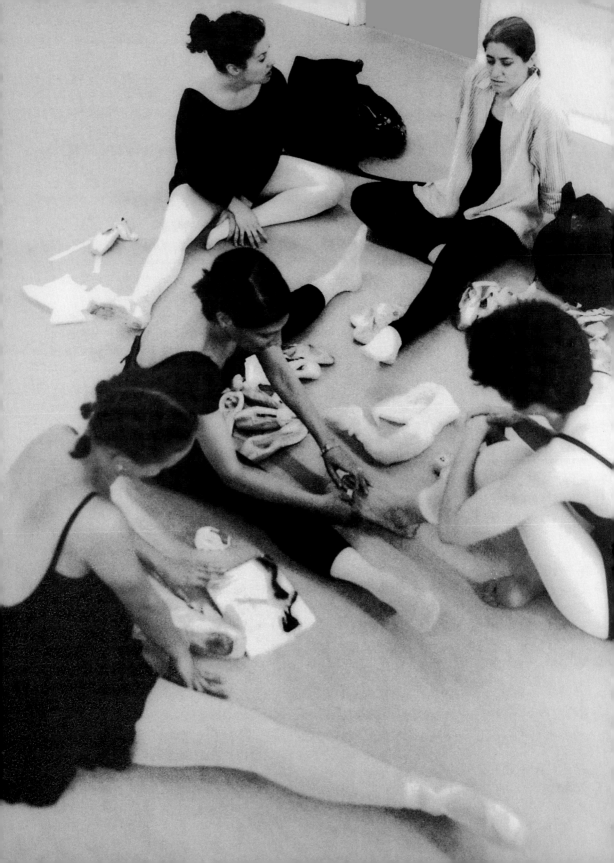

8

Pointe Work: How far can an adult beginner go?

MOST ADULT BEGINNERS don't even think about *pointe* work. Some may have been scared off because they didn't want to dance on their toes. Most adults don't ever try. If you're the exception, be prepared: *Pointe* class is very serious, very difficult, guaranteed to ruin your pedicure, and very satisfying. It may even be a dream come true, even if you only hold the barre with both hands and just do *relevés*. One Joffrey School adult beginner, when trying on her first *pointe* shoes, was overjoyed. "At my age, I never even considered that I ever could or ever would work *en pointe*. Just looking at the shoes and standing up in them would have been enough!"

We wish we could say that you can go as far with ballet as your inclination and desire take you. But, as in any endeavor, people have different abilities. Your ballet progress will be determined both by factors you can control (how often you come to class) and those you can't (body type and "talent"). It's why some adult beginners take to ballet and progress quickly, while others, who love it as much, don't. Fortunately, though, everyone and every body can benefit from ballet. You don't need to "graduate" to more advanced classes and you certainly don't need to dance *en pointe*.

For those adults who do go on to *pointe* work, it is, without question, another dimension of ballet. "I've attended ballet performances for years, of course, but all of a sudden, it hit me that everything on stage isn't done in soft shoes the way we practice in class, but all *en pointe*," one adult student marveled. "It was like a revelation, another world."

Pointe is what separates ballet from other dance forms; it's what gives ballet its special magic. For some adult students, *pointe* is the most tangible measure of their success. You've developed your skills to a recognizable level, and *pointe* work is your reward. It's also your opportunity to become physically stronger, more pulled up, and technically cleaner.

So, how far can an adult beginner go? Maybe all the way to *pointe* class. But only maybe. For some adults, *pointe* is a very valid goal, and truly an achievement to be proud of. If you are realistic and bear in mind that your *pointe* class won't lead to a professional career, you should be able to take great pride in what you've accomplished and enjoy the totality of your ballet experience.

P O I N T E   W O R K :
A   R E A L I T Y   C H E C K

If *pointe* is your goal, we advise keeping it a flexible one. Do you want to be able to dance *Giselle?* Or execute 32 *fouettés?* Or would you be satisfied to be able to do the barre exercises *en pointe?* (No small achievement, by the way.) One Joffrey adult beginner told us she only wanted to walk across the floor in her *pointe* shoes and feel like she was barefoot.

Other things to know before you get your hopes set on *pointe* work: It's an expensive hobby. Unless you're prepared to replace *pointe* shoes as necessary (at more than $50 a pair), don't consider it. But you can't work on shoes that are "dead"; i.e., when the *pointe* has soft spots and the shank has weakened to the degree that it offers no support. Remember, the adult body doesn't heal after an

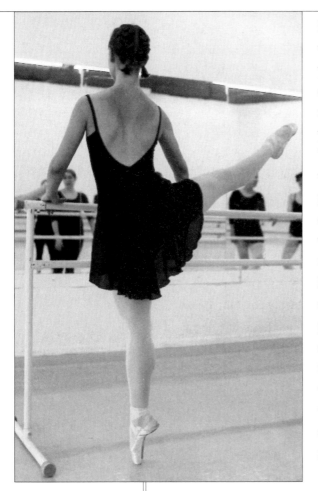

injury as well as it once did. *Pointe* work also may not be in the cards if you've got bunions or if your feet aren't shaped right for *pointe*. (No matter how competent you become in your ballet class, if your feet are "wrong," you may not want to deal with the discomfort. And "minor" problems can graduate very quickly to disasters!) Plus, it should be taken up with caution and only with your doctor's blessing if you've got knee problems (such as very bad arthritis or tendinitis) or back injuries (a sacroiliac or pelvic bones that are out of alignment, or weak abdominals and back muscles) that are causing you problems. Adults with poor circulation, bad varicose veins, and/or diabetes should also check with their doctors because of the friction and tightness of *pointe* shoes.

ADULT *POINTE* WORK AND "THE FANTASY"

With all of the above warnings and precautions, are you still intrigued by *pointe* work? There's no question that there's a mystique about it. For many adults, it goes back to childhood . . . slipping their feet into those elegant, beribboned pink satin *pointe* shoes does seem to be every little girl's dream. One Joffrey School faculty member remembers desperately wanting a pair of *pointe* shoes as a child, not necessarily to dance in, but just to own. "I was ten years old when I got them and they were wrapped up in pink tissue paper," she recalls. "I unwrapped them, slipped them on, and just pranced around the room." Emily, a Joffrey School adult beginner who returned to ballet in her late thirties, actually saved her first childhood *pointe* shoes—now moth-eaten and worn—a reminder of her first, early exploits. "I never really liked ballet class," she confesses. "I was too shy. But the special ritual of getting to wear real *pointe* shoes—tying up the ribbons, wrapping your toes in lambswool—was something else entirely."

For the adult who does advance to the level at which *pointe* is a viable option, taking a special adult *pointe* class, with a special teacher, can be a joy. (Classes with serious pre-professional dancers or students young enough to be their children won't meet the needs of the adult; the class will be structured differently and the adult will be competing unfairly for attention and correction.) First of all, there's the satisfaction (they said it couldn't be done!). Then, there's the pure, unadulterated delight and fulfillment—understanding physically the rationale for all the years of corrections and study. *Pointe* is the reason you've been admonished to pull up, to turn out, to straighten your legs: Suddenly, everything makes sense! When you're wearing *pointe* shoes, you don't have to be reminded to pull up, you feel it; it's obvious and natural. You suddenly understand turnout, too. Plus, there's the feeling of being so light that only your toes are touching the floor, all because you've got these wonderful pink things on your feet.

Is *Pointe* work for You?

While some teachers may suggest the challenge of *pointe* to adults who become proficient in class, most ballet teachers won't tell you when or if you're ready to go *en pointe*. Children who persevere with the study of ballet are expected to advance to *pointe*; adults generally are not expected to go that far and aren't encouraged to even consider it. The degree of expertise *pointe* requires, its potential for injury, the lack of adult beginner *pointe* classes all contribute to *pointe* not being considered a realistic or appropriate adult goal.

So how do you know if *pointe* work is for you? If there's ballet in your background—as a child, a teenager, a young adult—*pointe* may very well be an option. This is the one situation in which the adult who has had previous training has an advantage over those who have never studied before. Strength is a definite prerequisite. You need strong feet, calves, hips, and abdominals for *pointe*. (That's one of the reasons behind all the strengthening floorwork and exercises in class in the *Ballet-Fit* Workout.) Contrary to what many children think when they begin *pointe* at ages 10, 11, or 12, the *pointe* shoe doesn't hold you up. It's your foot, supported by your legs, supported by your middle. And it's not simply the challenge of staying up on your *pointe;* that's easy. It's going from the flat to the *pointe* and coming down on one foot as well as two. So, again, you have to be strong.

You need to have achieved a measure of competence in class, at the barre and in center, because whatever technical weaknesses you have will be exaggerated *en pointe*. Sickling your foot, for example, becomes more than just unattractive; it becomes dangerous. In *pointe* shoes, you can actually fracture the bones of your toes, foot, or ankle, if you're not turned out (turnout is what gives you the widest possible base of support for your trunk to balance over your feet). If you're not pulled up out of your shoes, you'll be putting too much weight on the shoes, and you won't be able to handle the physical demands of *pointe* work. Remember, you have to dance on your *pointes,* not just climb up there.

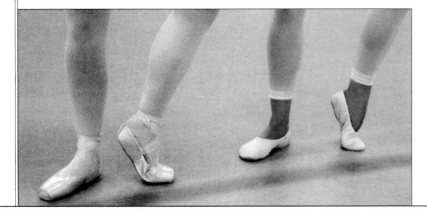

You need to take ballet classes on a regular basis. An adult who aspires to *pointe* should attend class no fewer than three times a week for a couple of years. If you're a regular (every day preferably), you may be ready for the challenge of *pointe*.

All of the above conditions notwithstanding, the shape of your foot has a lot to do with whether or not *pointe* work is for you, too. A squarish foot with short toes that are all approximately the same length is ideal for *pointe* work because the dancer's weight can be supported by a broader base. A long, narrow foot or one with disproportionate toes, like a protruding big or second toe, can be difficult to fit (although in the professional world, there have been notable exceptions). Other anatomical factors to consider: a very flexible foot with a high arch, which points easily, may look beautiful in *pointe* shoes, but because of its greater flexibility, it may not be as strong or easy to control, and may be prone to injuries like sprains, tendinitis, and dislocations.

Certain injuries and preexisting conditions make *pointe* work difficult, if not impossible. For example, if you have serious bunion problems or hammertoes, don't mess around with *pointe* shoes; they will be too painful and possibly damaging. Ditto for old knee or ankle and foot injuries. (We recommend that you check with your doctor before you stake out *pointe* as your ballet goal.) If you're not thin—if, in fact, you're as little as 8 to 10 pounds over your fighting weight—this is a good excuse to lose a little. Your family doctor may not know about the requirements for *pointe* work, but if you know a doctor who specializes in dance-related health issues (or who even has a background in dance), you may want to consult him or her before you consider an adult *pointe* class.

EIGHT-POINT CHECKLIST: YOU MAY BE READY FOR *POINTE* IF . . .

——— you are taking classes every day—or no fewer than three times a week—and have been for the past two years.

——— you are physically strong—your feet, your legs, your abdominals. While you don't have to be in performance shape, you really can't be overweight—not even 10 pounds. Remember, *en pointe,* all your weight, which is usually distributed on about eight inches of foot, is balanced on a little more than a single square inch!

——— you are able to articulate your feet. This is important because *pointe* shoes are not as responsive as soft shoes. By "articulate" we mean using your feet like hands, in *tendus,* in *frappés,* in everything.

——— you are capable of executing the ballet basics with ease and competence and are learning more advanced vocabulary. You should be able to execute at least a single *pirouette* in center.

——— you know how to place your weight, meaning when you're *en relevé,* you can hit your balance and hold it.

——— you are competent at *pointe* preparation exercises in center like *pas de bourrée, échappé,* and *passé relevé.*

——— you have developed a soft and elastic *plié* and you know how to use it.

——— you have reached a level where you no longer have trouble remembering combinations.

In addition to all of the above, the language of ballet should be automatic to you. Because the shoes themselves can be so distracting, if the vocabulary is not already in your muscles, you won't be able to follow. Sometimes, students just can't focus on what comes next when they've got these "things" on their feet! They're brandnew, they're not broken in (and presumably no one has told you to break them in, but we will, see page 211), they weigh a ton, they feel awful and awkward. So much for the fantasy . . .

see page 211

PRETTY SHOES, UGLY FEET

Even with all precautions taken, *pointe* work will probably cause your feet to blister. When you've blistered often enough, you may develop a callus or bump (eventually, your toes will stop blistering because the bump will protect them). Don't try to get rid of the bumps until you've stopped working *en pointe*.

Other consequences of *pointe* work: Don't be surprised if your nails show considerable wear and tear from pressure: bruising and discoloration, thickening, ridges or cracks (sometimes they even break off!). Take pride in your ugly feet—they are feet that work. When you stop working *en pointe*, after a time, they should return to their previous state of pristine beauty. One Joffrey School faculty member said it took five years for her feet to return to their normal state, but she was wearing *pointe* shoes every day and taking seventeen classes a week!

INSIDER'S TIP

Prepare your feet for *pointe* by *not* having a pedicure. You will need all the lumps and bumps and calluses you've developed in your regular class (plus your nail polish will be vulnerable to abrasion and chipping, so it's practically a waste, anyway). In addition, we advise you to keep your toenails short, but not so short that the tender skin under the nail is exposed. Bottom line: Your feet will not be as beautiful without shoes as they will be with the shoes on.

THE JOFFREY BALLET SCHOOL'S BALLET-FIT

Most *pointe* shoes have drawstrings, although some, like Russian-made shoes, don't. Instead, they have a deep, V-shaped vamp. Dancers generally sew fabric on the inside of the vamp to draw the vamp together, closing the V and tailoring the shoe for a better fit.

BUYING *POINTE* SHOES

If you've gotten the go-ahead from your teacher to pursue *pointe* work and have found an appropriate class, your next step is to buy your *pointe* shoes—no small task. Do you buy them in the same place you bought your ballet slippers and leotard? (No, not if you bought those in your local hosiery shop.) Ask at your school or check the theater district in your city for dance-supply houses that cater to professional dancers. And expect to make more than one visit to more than one shop before you find the right shoe. If there are no appropriate shops in your area, you may even have to resort to mail order, which is doable, if not exactly ideal. How this usually works: You trace an outline of your foot and send it along with other requested information. See the *Ballet-Fit* Source Directory for a sampling of mail-order resources for shops. Also, if you have a foot that's hard to fit, you may have to have shoes custom-made (professionals do all the time), and it's not as expensive as you might think. Sometimes, too, there are sales at ballet-supply houses. One adult beginner's first pair of *pointe* shoes—bought brand-new but at half price—was a special order that was rejected for some reason that didn't affect the quality of the shoe.

We've seen lists describing the characteristics of various brands of *pointe* shoes: Capezio is the most widely available brand; Freed's *pointe* shoes are light and comfortable; Bloch's are strong. In the last decade, there's been such an explosion of new brands and types of shoes on the market, and there are so many variables (from the shape of your foot to what's available where you live), that we can't comfortably suggest one or even two particular brands as being most suitable for beginners. There are Australian shoes and Austrian shoes and English shoes. There are American shoes. In New York, we've heard good things about Russian-made shoes that some dancers like (they have the tiniest toe—barely the size of a quarter—and they make your feet look gorgeous). But *pointe* shoes are handmade, and as with soft ballet shoes, there will be all sorts of variations in the sizing. Every maker, for example, has a different last, which has a different fit and feel. You have to sort them out—and try them on—yourselves. (Professional dancers use lots of different shoes—some are harder, some softer, some more broken in than others, since the choreography sometimes dictates the type of shoe they need to wear. If the choreography calls for a lot of jumps, for example, the dancer may want a softer shoe that responds to the foot better. If there are *fouettés* [a very demanding type of turn as in the 32 *fouettés* in the *Black Swan* variations], and the dancer will be *en pointe* constantly, she'll want a harder shoe.)

In general, beginners should look for shoes that have enough support through the shank and box, that are as comfortable as possible, and that flatter their feet (there are subtle variations which you'll notice in time). Heavier shoes with square boxes offer a larger surface on which to balance and may be preferable for beginners whose feet ususally aren't strong enough to handle lighter, more flexible shoes, or those with tinier *pointes*. The shoes should not be so stiff and heavy, however, that they prevent you from "feeling the floor," from making use of your *demi-pointe* position, and using your feet properly.

When you try on *pointe* shoes for the first time—or for the first time in twenty or thirty years—we only hope you get a knowledgeable and sympathetic salesperson. We've met some superbly informed salespeople, but we've also met more than our share of those who are clueless—and, while well-meaning, are downright misinformed about the particulars of *pointe*. Of course it can be helpful to bring someone knowledgeable with you, such as a more advanced student or your teacher. But if you've got to go it alone, arm yourself with as much solid information as possible.

How should *pointe* shoes feel? Probably nothing like what you imagine. They're not bedroom slippers, we concede, but they're far from ancient Chinese foot binding, either. They do need to be snug—much more constricting than your street shoes—although

PADDING AND TAPING

When you buy your *pointe* shoes, leave room at the toe for padding. Although some professionals tough it out with nothing at all, adult beginners are well advised to buy lambswool or any of the other types of padding. Padding protects the toes and minimizes the rubbing of the skin against the shoe, but still allows the dancer to feel the floor. Avoid overthick plastic or sponge pads as well as fur pads which can make the feet perspire.

If you choose lambswool (our preference), choose the fluffy, soft kind, wrap it around your toes where they are most likely to hurt (typical trouble spots include the big toe, the little toe, the knuckles and the tips of the toes). If you use too much though, the shoes will be too tight; they'll hurt. Besides, there shouldn't be room for that much padding, if there is, you've bought the wrong shoe size.

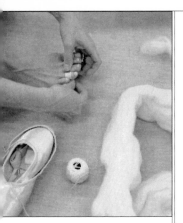

Later, as you progress, you may discover you like tissues in your shoe, paper towels, or other variations.

The other thing that dancers and dance students do is tape their toes, which provides even more protection. Adhesive tape is the tape of choice; fold it back so the adhesive doesn't touch your skin. Wrap your toes where the shoes tend to rub most (often over the toes' knuckles). Don't wrap the tape too tightly, though; when you're working *en pointe*, your feet will swell and the tape can feel like a tourniquet and cause blisters. You may prefer to use Band-Aids, because they provide another cushion.

not so snug that your toes curl up. (Your toes should almost reach the end of the shoe, with some room leftover—but not much—for lambswool.) All *pointe* shoes, by the way, are pink, except those that are dyed black or other colors for special performances. Elastics come with the shoe; matching ribbons are usually purchased at the store, but both need to be sewn on.

When you try on *pointe* shoes for the first time, don't expect to be able to walk around in them. Not only are they not broken in, but until the elastics are sewn on, the backs will flap off when you walk. You should be able to stand in them, however, and to *relevé*. Many stores have a bit of wooden floor and a barre so prospective *pointe* shoe buyers can waddle over and test them out.

As with any other pair of shoes, it's important how they feel and fit, flat. There should be minimal creasing at the toe and across the top of the shoes. They shouldn't twist or gap (either flat or in *relevé*). Your longest toes should barely graze the top of the shoe, and your foot should be approximately the same as the shoe length, with the smallest amount left over for lambswool or very light padding (see the sidebar). If you have long toes, you'll want a deep vamp to support the toes as much as possible, but not too deep, which can make it difficult to get "over the *pointe*"; that is, to achieve a full *pointe* position. Note: *En pointe*, when the ankle is in line with the toe, is called "getting over the *pointe.*" The knee, the ankle, and the toe should all be in alignment.

PREPARING POINTE SHOES

Just as there is a ritual to buying *pointe* shoes, there's also a ritual to preparing them. But don't do anything until you've asked your teacher to okay the fit. (That's only your first pair, however. After that you'll have a good idea of how they should fit and what to look for, although your teacher is always a good resource and may even have a few tricks of her own to show you.)

After you've purchased your shoes, brought them into class,

Although you usually buy ribbons when you buy your *pointe* shoes, there's no reason why you can't also pick up appropriate ribbon at your local notions or sewing store, where you can select the thickness, quality, and type (satin is most popular although grosgrain ribbon or bias or binding tape have the advantage of not slipping). For classroom use, dancers use whatever ribbons they happen to have on hand. While you're at your local notions store, pick up some heavy, darning-quality thread for sewing on the ribbons—it's stronger. Some dancers also use dental floss, but we doubt that the rigors of an adult beginner *pointe* class equal those of a three-hour performance!

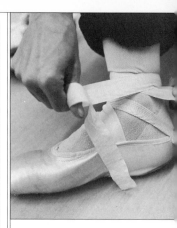

TYING RIBBONS CORRECTLY

There is a particular way that *pointe* shoe ribbons are tied: Put your foot flat on the floor, fully flexed. Cross the ribbon in front of the ankle, then cross it behind the ankle, then wrap it around the front of the leg, one ribbon on top of the other, knotting both ends tightly, on the inside of the ankle, right above the ankle bone. Tuck the knot neatly underneath the ribbon in the hollow of the ankle. Never tie your shoes with a bow. It's unprofessional.

and had your teacher check the fit, the first part of the ritual is to sew on the elastics and ribbon. Elastics, which help to hold the back of the shoe on, are available in different widths, and when you purchase your shoes, you should be asked what width you prefer (we find wider elastics hold better and tend not to "cut"). If you're not asked, *tell* the salesperson what you want. Sew them on either side of the back seam of the shoe, on the outside, not the inside (because the shoes are so snug, if they were sewn inside they would chafe your foot). Don't sew a loop of elastic on the back. It may seem like to a good idea to slip the ribbon into, but it presses against the Achilles tendon.

There are several schools of thought about *pointe* shoe ribbons. The party line has you cutting the ribbon in half (it comes in one piece, enough for two shoes), folding down the shoe's back and sewing the ribbon at that point. By sewing the ribbon farther back on the shoe, more foot shows and the eyes of the audience aren't drawn to the ribbon.

There's nothing wrong with this method for performers, but we think it's better to sew the ribbon where it does you, the adult beginner, the most good. Your foot may not look better, but we believe it will be more effective if you sew it closer to the middle

If you need help tying ribbons the first time, ask your teacher or a more experienced student to show you how to tie your shoes; there is an art to it. Don't be embarrassed about asking for help (which is preferable to showing up in class with your ribbons laced up to your knees and finished off with a great big bow!). In ballet class, it's far tackier to pretend that you're an insider when you're not than to be honest about who you are.

BALLET-FIT TIP

Tying your *pointe* shoe ribbons may come out neater if you do it one ribbon at a time. You may also have read somewhere that performers sew the knot so that the ribbons don't unravel on stage. Don't waste time doing this; in class, you have the option of sitting down and retying your shoe. You may also have read somewhere in ballet lore about darning the *pointe* of your shoes to cushion the *pointe* and make them last longer and to prevent slipping on stage, but we don't personally know anyone who still does that.

seam of the shoe (for some people, that's a spot that holds better and makes your foot look more arched). So experiment by pinning the ribbon in place before you sew it on.

Ribbons are sewn on the inside of the shoe. Sew them securely but not so well so that you can't pick out the stitches to remove the ribbon when your shoes wear out. Ribbons are routinely removed by dance students and professionals, frugal and not so, so they can be washed and reused; your shoes may be "dead" after taking three one-hour classes, but the ribbons may still have plenty of life in them. We also suggest tucking the ribbons under when you sew—about an inch and half of ribbon will do it—in case you just want to cut the ribbons off your shoes in order to use them again.

In the old days, the unsewn end of the ribbon was hemmed to prevent unraveling. We recommend quickly passing the unsewn ribbon end through a flame, which will melt the end and accomplish the same purpose.

HOW LONG DO *POINTE* SHOES LAST?

We've said that *pointe* shoes don't last that long; in fact, on stage, they may wear out during a single performance, and several pairs of shoes may be necessary in the course of the evening. True. *Pointe* shoes are only made of strips of fabric and glue, put together in a way similar to *papier-mâché*. *Pointes* melt due to body heat and perspiration and shanks become too soft to support the dancer even in the course of a two-hour performance!

So how long can adult beginners expect their shoes to last? It depends on the adult, the shoe, and how many classes you're taking per week. If you attend a one-hour class *en pointe* per week, your shoes could last anywhere from three weeks to three months, a variable which has nothing to do with the price of the shoe (a more expensive shoe, in other words, may not be the longest lasting). There are now shoes coming on the market made of new, space-age materials, which may have a longer life. We'll see. But the classic kind do wear out.

What can you do with your old *pointe* shoes? Companies often sell the autographed *pointe* shoes of their stars in order to raise funds, but you can take the shank out and wear them for soft practice shoes (students often do this because they offer more resistance against the floor, and their feet get stronger faster; professionals, of course, tend to take all their classes *en pointe*). Or you can hang them on the wall for inspiration, or autograph them and give them to your friends, your mother, your boyfriend, or anyone else who told you it couldn't be done.

MAKING *POINTE* SHOES LAST

Dance students have lots of ways of squeezing an extra week or so out of their shoes, using Krylon (a fixative for pastels), polyurethane, or acrylic floor wax. Make sure you use these substances on the *inside* of the shoe to avoid making the *pointe* too slippery. Some dancers reinforce the shoes' soles (to keep the shank strong) with polyurethane and acrylic floor wax, too. Ask some of the more experienced students in your class for their secrets.

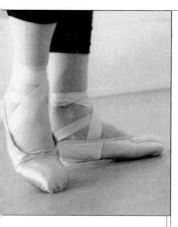

It's also a good idea to gently "arch" the shoe, to help make it more supple and flexible, taking care not to break the shank. Advanced dancers often deliberately break the shank or buy shoes with a half or three-quarter shank, but beginners need the support of a full shank.

BREAKING THEM IN

Although you may be bursting with pride at the sight of your precious, bright and shiny, new pink shoes, you are going to have to break them in which, you may have heard, calls for banging them on the floor, slamming them in a door and all sorts of other disconcerting things. Professional dancers do this; you're not going to.

The real story: As a beginner you're going to need all the support the shoe can offer you. Dancing or even just taking class on brand-new shoes can be uncomfortable and distracting, but you don't want to wear them out before you've even danced in them. Here's what to do:

1. Begin by putting the shoes on. Then, saturate a cotton ball with rubbing alcohol.

2. Look at your feet. Where do the shoes hurt? Around the big toe? Across the knuckles? The little toe? With your foot in the shoe, saturate the pink satin with the alcohol on all the tight places. Many dancers will soften the shoe around the joint of the big toe and the little toe (this part of the shoe is called the wings).

3. Next, while the shoe is still wet, walk around on *demi-pointe,* letting the alcohol soften the shoes, stretching it where you need it to be more flexible, till it eventually dries in the shape of your foot (approximately 5 to 10 minutes). You can also put a little alcohol on the sole of the shoe, right under the arch to increase its flexibility, although that stiffness will work itself out as you use the shoe.

As you go through this process, take care not to soak or even splash alcohol on the *pointe* of the shoe, as the alcohol can soften it. Some beginners need the wings for support; others (people with shorter toes, for instance) just find them abrasive and will use alcohol there). Eventually, as you wear the shoe, they'll just melt from the heat of your foot and perspiration.

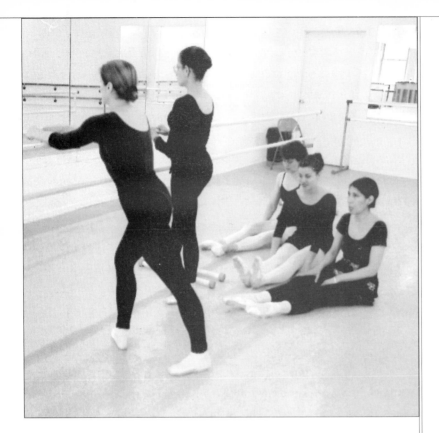

WHAT TO EXPECT IN *POINTE* CLASS

Now that you've got your *pointe* shoes—and prepared them—perhaps you're wondering how your beginner *pointe* class will differ from the ballet class you're used to?

Beginner *pointe* class won't be unfamiliar to you, and if the class is well designed, it should be challenging but not demanding.

Some teachers simply conduct their regular beginner technique class but ask for *relevé en pointe*. Others modify the basic barre, emphasizing *demi-plié* and footwork like *tendu, battement tendu jeté,* and *ronds de jambe* and adding special exercises designed for *pointe* work like *échappé,* springing up and rolling

INSIDER'S TIP

A good way to approach *pointe* for adults is to speak to your teacher about doing five minutes of *pointe* after your regular technique class, and gradually working yourself up to taking an entire class *en pointe*. If your school doesn't offer an adult beginner *pointe* class, your teacher might even suggest that you take your regular class (or part of it) in *pointe* shoes.

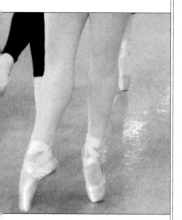

down in all positions, and *pas de bourrée*. You may start out, for example, with *demi-plié* combinations, often facing the barre, but there will be more emphasis on rolling through the foot in order to strenghten the foot and learn how to use the shoes. Center work, mercifully, will be short: It could be a *piqué* combination or sometimes just walking across the floor, on the diagonal, *en pointe*. And since all of this is far from natural, you'll spend quite a bit of time learning how to get up on your toes (staying up is not the problem, it's getting there that's the trick).

Part of the class, of course, involves simply getting used to the shoes, which start out clumsy and awkward. Pink satin notwithstanding, they are not beautiful in and of themselves; it's up to you to make them beautiful and make them work, which is what the class is all about. Some teachers even start their beginner *pointe* classes without shoes, with pointing and flexing exercises, followed by a *tendu* combination. It's only then that everyone puts on her shoes together (often you have to work up to wearing your *pointe* shoes for the whole class). But bear with it. As one teacher put it, tongue in cheek: "By the end of the *pliés* your feet will be numb and you won't feel a thing."

One question that adult beginners often ask is how it can be possible to "feel the floor"—a ballet directive—with their feet so encased? This is why *pointe* work is difficult: You have to *learn* how to feel the floor. That's why the Joffrey School technique stresses articulation of the feet as part of *pointe* preparation. It's only when you put on hard shoes for the first time that you know what you're up against. By the way, some people call them hard shoes or blocked shoes but never toe shoes; that's a layperson's term. And in the class or studio, it's always *en pointe*, never "on toe." Note: Don't be surprised if all of a sudden you see someone in your *pointe* class do something very beautiful and very advanced. There may well be quite a few people in class who have some *pointe* background but haven't done it in ten years. Or there may simply be no other class available for them to take.

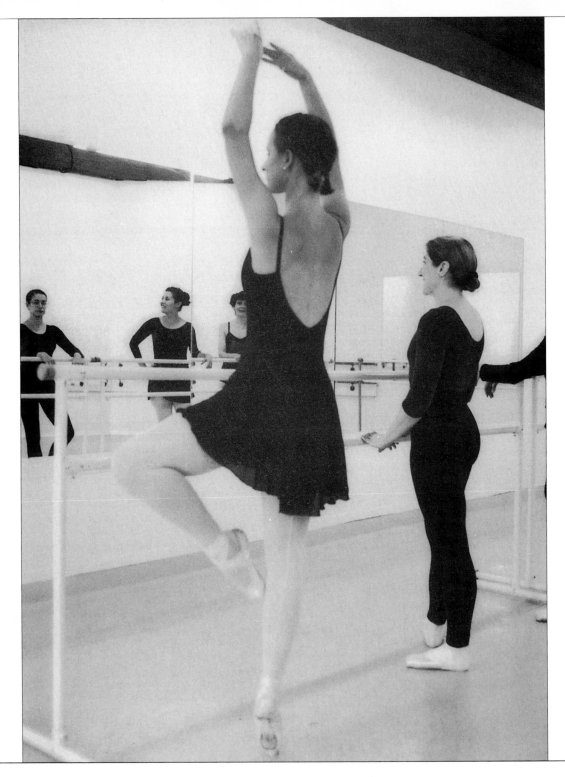

THE JOFFREY BALLET SCHOOL'S BALLET-FIT

Part of the fun and fantasy of ballet is putting on your first *pointe* shoes, or your first *pointe* shoes since you were a kid. "It truly gave me a different perspective about what actually goes on on stage, and what the students in the more advanced classes are feeling," one adult beginner wrote. Once you start doing a little *pointe* work, it helps your technique.

You have to pull up, you have to use your feet, you have to use your *plié,* you have to use your turnout as much as you are physically able to. If you don't, you can't stand up. Your *pointe* class and your regular technique class reinforce each other. The best preparation for *pointe* is consistent technique classes, and what you learn in *pointe* class, you will carry over to your regular classes. You can certainly consider *pointe* a milestone, although not doing *pointe* for whatever reason shouldn't spoil the pleasure you derive from your regular technique classes; it certainly won't diminish the fitness benefits.

Finally, in your beginner *pointe* class, expect all the adults to have shoes that are shiny and new, and ribbons that look a bit untidy. Everyone will be uncomfortable . . . and proud . . . and excited . . . and be having a wonderful time. Good luck!

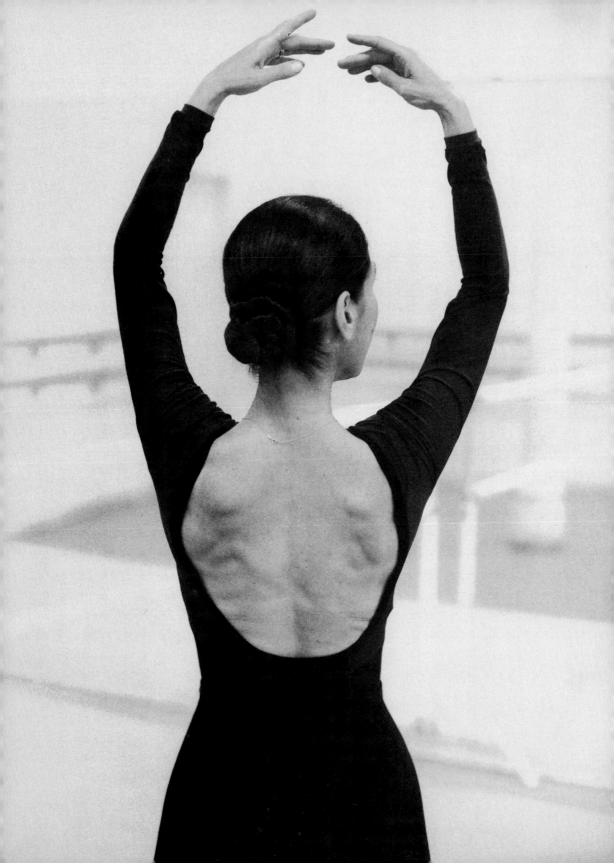

9

$\mathcal{A}$nswers to Commonly Asked Adult Ballet Questions

$\sim$

Do I need to take a certain amount of ballet classes a week to benefit?

Frankly, if you want to progress quickly, a once-a-week ballet class will not be enough. You—and your body—won't remember from week to week. To maximize the body sculpting benefits of ballet, the more classes you take, the faster you'll see and feel the effects. If progress is your goal, try to follow up your ballet class with some aerobic activity three to five times per week and do the floor exercises three times a week as well. That's not to say you won't learn if you do less. You will, but at a slower rate. But if you're patient, the results will come, no matter how infrequently you work. Keep in mind, you're not limited to just three classes a week; take as many as your schedule allows. Some adults feel best when they've had a daily ballet workout while others have been known to take as many classes as a young dancer in training. There are also specific exercise techniques taught by and for dancers (Pilates comes to mind), which could be an option for you.

I'm always traveling. If I can't take ballet classes on a regular basis, does it make any sense to take a class only now and then?

We're not going to say no. Many of our adult students have jobs or lifestyles that involve extensive travel, and they take whichever classes work into their schedules. They also travel with favorite audiotapes and try to give themselves a ballet workout as often as they can.

If you need to, you can record your class (ask your teacher and the pianist first), or you can take notes during or after class so you won't have to struggle to remember the sequence of the exercises. While we're traveling, we usually like to do the *Ballet-Fit* Warm-up and a quick barre—*pliés, tendus, battements, jetés, ronds des jambes,* and *fondus*—floor exercises, and explore the fitness facilities wherever we're staying.

But there's no need to be compulsive in order to keep fit. If you're on vacation, you're probably walking more than usual, climbing stairs or hills, swimming, or skiing. If you're on business, you're probably under pressure and don't need to feel guilty about not doing everything. When you return, take your regular class, remembering that your goals are fitness and relaxation, not preparing for your stage debut.

I studied ballet as a child, but I remember doing some things differently. Was I taught badly then or now?

Most likely, when you were a child you were taught according to the method most popular at that time in your community, and now as an adult, you are taught according to the method most popular at this time in your community. In other words, styles change. For example, some of us remember being taught that the hands should be held as if they were bunches of grapes—very drippy-looking. Nothing could be farther from what is taught today, when we try to hold the hands and arms with strength and energy. Which is right? In the context of ballet history, both are, or were. What you're remembering, most likely, are the differences between the wrapped foot and the flexed foot for *frappés;* the height of the arm in *arabesque*—all differences that are legitimate. What is preferable depends on your teacher. The short answer: You may well have been taught badly (teachers vary, and there really isn't a governing body that offers credentials to all ballet teachers), but more likely what you're remembering reflects differences in style.

I tried ballet once and really hated it. Was it my fault or what?

Not everyone takes to ballet, any more than everyone likes fencing or tennis or skiing. The aesthetic component sets it apart from other demanding physical activities. Form is essential, and learning the form takes time. If you want a quick fix, ballet probably isn't for you.

But ballet also comes with a lot of baggage. Children's teachers are not always as sensitive as they should be, and even teachers of adults may not always be gracious. You may have had a bad experience. But try it again (you're obviously intrigued). Not everyone likes caviar the first time they try it either.

Why do we value being "professional," when we're not professionals and don't aspire to be?

Your teacher is a professional. Dancers study for many years, with seriousness and devotion, often leaving other talents and interests behind. It's a courtesy and great compliment to you, the adult beginner, to be treated as an aspiring "professional," even if it means reminding you to tuck in the drawstrings on your shoes and put your hair up, to be quiet in class, and take turns going across the floor.

In addition, keep in mind that teachers are awed by their adult students' abilities and accomplishments in the "real" world. That's

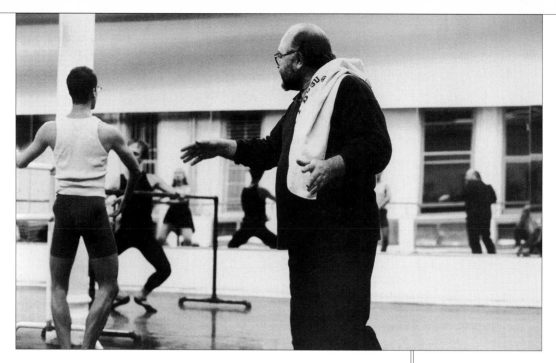

why they expect you to honor theirs. Your presence in class is the first sign of respect. Your willingness to adapt to the demands of the history, tradition, and customs of ballet indicates your willingness to learn and become part of the ballet world, even if you're taking one class a week.

Help! My teacher hates me—and it's the only ballet class in my town. What can I do?

What could you possibly have done to make the teacher hate you? We assume, of course, that you don't argue with the teacher or show up wearing purple Spandex and heavy perfume!

Don't let the infantilizing aspects of ballet class get to you. You can speak with your teacher privately to sort out what the problem is; or simply take your class, conduct yourself appropriately, do your best—and ignore it. Keep in mind that ballet teachers are not trained primarily as teachers and may not always be entirely objective. It may be the teacher's problem, not yours.

What's the benefit of private classes?

Private class can be tricky. Sometimes, if it's only a matter of getting more attention, they can be a waste of your time and a lot of your money, because learning ballet is based on repetition. Other times, they may be helpful; i.e., when you've hit a plateau and can't seem to progress no matter how hard you work. Private classes can also be valuable when you've advanced beyond your class and may even be ready to start *pointe,* but classes aren't open to you at your new level; or if you've gotten to a stage where you want to learn some choreography (at these times, studying individually with a teacher is a reward for work well done). But most often, ballet is best pursued in a class with other students at your level, so you can learn from their mistakes as well as your own. We find that the dynamics of a class approximate the dynamics of the stage.

I've had recent surgery. Should I let my teacher know, and if so, when?

We urge you to tell your teacher anything—no matter how personal—that relates to your ability to function in class: This includes injuries, illnesses, pregnancy, extended vacations, medications (even antidepressants), all of which may change how you work in class. If your teacher is not made aware of a condition that makes you vulnerable, you could hurt yourself. The goal in teaching adults is not merely fitness, but fitness without injury.

We know there aren't a lot of opportunities to speak privately with your teacher, so if you have to, leave your teacher a note (with your phone number if necessary). This is the one obligation you have to yourself, your teacher, and your school.

Other personal matters, like an emotional crisis (which, we know, may certainly affect your performance in class), may not be appropriate to share; that's up to you.

My beginner class seems to consist of *pliés* and *tendus* and a few little jumps at the end. Why do we have to do the same things over and over?

It's essential to learn the basics and to learn them well. Ballet is primarily technique, and classes are—or should be—graded; this means that teachers systematically introduce ballet placement and basic vocabulary ("steps") and reinforce what they've taught by repetition. Since ballet steps build one on another, it's important to learn these basics and to learn them well, before progressing to more difficult steps. Adult students may get impatient but should realize that, unlike academic subjects, ballet exercises are not just learned, they are honed and perfected to the utmost degree, which in itself can be satisfying.

In other words, just because you've "done" *assemblé* in class last week, doesn't mean that you can now put it aside and learn *entrechats*. It's up to the teacher to present familiar material in interesting and challenging combinations so that each element gets better, quicker, and more beautiful.

The advanced ballet classes move so much more than my adult class, which seems static in comparison. When will we do more "steps"?

Ballet is movement, but it's movement with technique. Before a dancer can fly across the floor, he or she must be willing to undergo several years of *pliés* and *tendus,* stretching and strengthening the feet, the legs, and the whole body (advanced dancers usually start taking ballet at the age of eight, or even earlier in a program like the Joffrey School's preballet class). This means that by the time students have reached an intermediate or advanced class, they have perhaps five or more years of systematic training.

But the adult beginner can advance, too. There is no reason why an adult who takes two or more classes per week over the

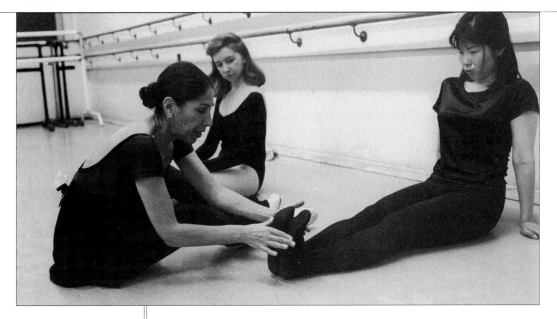

course of two years cannot learn more complex combinations at lively tempos. And again, some adults who started as beginners may even develop enough strength to start *pointe* work.

I come to class to exercise and relax, not because I want to dance. Why should I bother with center work if I really don't enjoy it?

Of course, you don't have to. And the truth is, center work is not essential for fitness (jumps may be valuable as aerobic exercise, but in ballet they aren't sustained long enough to provide substantial benefits). If fitness and relaxation are your goals—and the pressure of anticipating center is spoiling it for you—do what makes you happy as long as it's all right with your teacher.

On the other hand, take a look at the answer to the next question, which might convince you to give it a try.

I love the barre and floor exercises in my class, but I feel uncomfortable doing center. I don't want to stop coming to class, but I'm starting to feel embarrassed about "ducking out." Do I have to do it?

As we said to the reader previously, you don't have to take center if you don't want to. But we urge you to keep at it, keeping in mind that students usually advance much quicker at the barre than they do in center. It's hard!

For many students, center is the most pleasurable part of the class; it's when you put into practice what you've learned at the barre and what you've been strengthening your body for. Plus, it's the most like dancing.

Because adults do get frustrated by the difficulty of center work, we believe that center needs to be taught slowly; some adults pick up movement naturally, some don't. Movement—the essence of dance—comes from inside, and in ballet class we have to be encouraged to allow ourselves to move.

Finally, adults who are competitive in their daily lives tend to bring that sense of competition to center work as well (if they feel they're not progressing as fast as they should, their anxieties and inadequacies surface—which they shouldn't). Try to keep in mind that ballet class is noncompetitive and do what you want to do about center . . . but we think you're missing out.

I'm really busy. I can't be on someone else's schedule. How can I fit a ballet class into my life?

If you're serious about wanting to stay fit, you have to make time for it, and that may require a little schedule juggling if it's not part of your day to start with. Some people get up early in the morning; others catch a class on their lunch hour; still others fit a class in on their way home from work in the evening. You may have to do your *pliés* while watching the evening news.

In addition, keep in mind that you needn't take the same class every week. Many adults in urban areas wind up taking different classes, given at different times, at different schools, and creating a schedule of their own; one school may offer evening classes for adults, another may have a Saturday morning class that fits perfectly into your life. Tailor your schedule to your needs, supplementing with videos or audios, or the *Ballet-Fit* Workout, which you can do at home, on your own schedule, whenever you like.

Are there opportunities for adults to perform (realistically)?

Ballet is a performing art, not simply a fitness technique, and to some degree, every class can be seen as a performance in which you are expected to do your best. At some level of training, however, adults may have a desire to perform on stage.

We want to stress that while a professional career is unlikely, that's not the end of it. There are community groups, local performances by dance schools that require well-trained adults (as in *The Nutcracker*) and other nonprofessional options.

Don't be too shy to explore such opportunities with your teacher; after all, your desire to perform reflects positively on his or her teaching. And don't discount the opportunity to learn to teach, yourself. Schools with heavy schedules of children's and

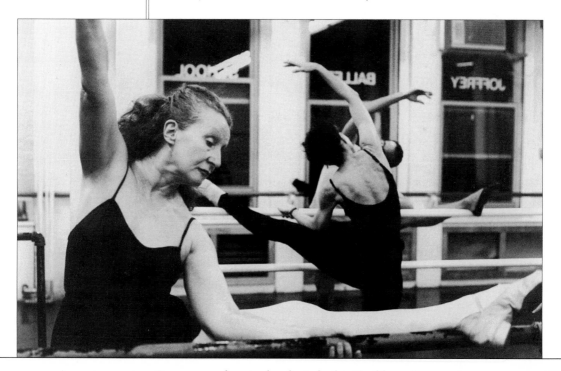

adult classes often welcome teaching assistants, which is a good way to start.

I love ballet. I know I'm not going to be a professional dancer, but I really want to make dance my life. Is this silly?

Not at all. It's never too late to pursue something you love, as long as you can be realistic about it. Even though you're unlikely to be able to perform professionally in ballet, there may be opportunities for you in other dance disciplines, like modern dance or jazz, or ballroom dancing, where training can begin in your twenties (and where your ballet experience can be put to good use).

In addition, there's more to the dance world than performing. Why not consider other related areas of theater crafts such as costume, lighting, scenery, or set design and manufacture. You can research dance history and teach; volunteer to assist with children's ballet classes; or pursue a career in dance administration, dance pedagogy, dance therapy, or arts management if you're willing to take graduate-level courses. One of our adult ballet students is a dance videographer. The possibilities are almost endless (see the *Ballet-Fit* Source Directory for university programs that may give you some ideas).

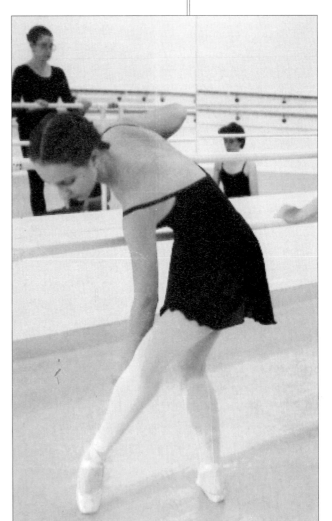

Are jazz, modern dance, tap, flamenco, and other dance forms a good complement to ballet?

These days, the lines dividing dance forms are fading, so take whatever form of dance appeals to you. Career-oriented ballet students are studying jazz, tap, modern, and ethnic dance, and doing cartwheels across the floor. Ballet companies are staging productions that look like rock videos; ballet choreographers are creating dances on Broadway, while modern choreographers are finding work with ballet companies. We're in favor of dance, period.

How do I know when I've advanced enough to go on to a harder class?

If only it were as easy as being promoted from fourth grade to fifth! Under the Royal Academy of Dancing (RAD) system, students are required to complete a curriculum before moving up. But for the vast majority of adult beginners, moving to a more advanced class depends on whether or not one is available. In a school or studio where graded classes are offered, you might want to observe the next level and try it when you feel ready. (You'll know you're in the right class if you can't quite keep up—but if you're totally lost beginning with *pliés,* wait another few months before you try again.) Objectively, if you can complete your present class with relative ease and can do a double *pirouette* and 16 *entrechat quatres* or *royales,* you're probably ready to advance.

My ballet school asked me to sign a release. What does it mean?

The studio wants to avoid paying you damages if you get hurt. Although a waiver or release doesn't necessarily preclude you from suing the school for gross negligence, it's a first step toward reducing their liability for injuries. Our lawyer friends tell us that when you dance or skate or lift weights or go riding at a riding stable, you "assume the risk" of injury, and you've got a heavy burden of proof that the school (or ice rink, gym, or stable) was at fault. Common sense tells you to watch for slippery or sticky floors, staircases without handrails and the like, and report to the administration any condition that, in your judgment, could be dangerous.

I was a really serious ballet student when I was a teenager (I even auditioned for dance jobs). What should I expect if I come back to an adult class?

Expect to be an adult beginner. Don't expect to look the way you did when you were 18, or to dance the way you did when you were 18 (you may remember what to do intellectually, but your muscles will complain!), but do expect to experience all the feelings you had as a young dancer. This was the situation in one Joffrey School adult class in which a young woman burst into tears of frustration after class (she explained that it was her first class since she was 18 and auditioning, and she was upset at how she looked and danced). Of course, in the adult class she was lovely, obviously well trained, and very competent, but she was also obviously not 18 anymore.

For some, returning to ballet as a nonprofessional may be a difficult transition, for others it can be profoundly positive. In fact, it's wonderful to know that ballet can still be part of your life. You may end up working more slowly than you once did, but you also may enjoy and appreciate it more.

I am an avid tennis player . . . rider . . . skier. How will these sports affect my ballet class?

As a recreational dancer, you should feel free to pursue all the physical activities you normally enjoy. In terms of overall fitness, you can only benefit. Serious dancers should bear in mind that most sports develop muscles that aren't compatible with ballet. For example, in tennis or skiing, you work in parallel *plié*—which is very different from ballet. But again, for the recreational dancer, taking ballet class two or three times a week, it shouldn't matter at all.

I don't know much about music but I like what I hear in class. How can I learn more?

Ask your teacher or accompanist (if your class has one) about the music you especially like. Then, check out your library or music store and find other music by the same composer. The liner notes can be a very helpful introduction to music analysis and music history.

The following are some traditional ballet favorites that may be familiar to you, and that can get your started: Tchaikovsky's *Swan Lake, Nutcracker,* or *Sleeping Beauty;* Prokofiev's *Romeo and Juliet;* Stravinsky's *Petroushka;* Glazunov's *Raymonda;* Adolphe Adam's *Giselle.* But we also urge you to go beyond the familiar; be open to

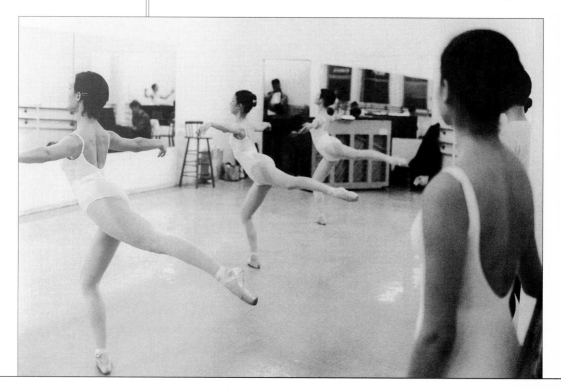

Answers to Commonly Asked Adult Ballet Questions

music that's new to you and don't limit yourself. Choreographers are now using modern classics like Cole Porter or George Gershwin, or even rock music, for ballet.

I'm obsessed. I eat, drink, and sleep my ballet class and am only happy when I'm in the ballet studio. It's taking over my life. What can I do?

This sounds pretty serious. Don't let ballet interfere with your real life. Lots of people get caught up in their fitness routines (one woman we know wouldn't schedule a vacation with her family for more than three days because she'd miss her three-hour daily workout). But ballet—or any fitness activity—shouldn't jeopardize your relationships, your job, or your health. If ballet is really what you want to do in life, consult the *Ballet-Fit* Source Directory for career opportunities.

ACKNOWLEDGMENTS

OUR SINCERE THANKS to the many people who participated in this book: foremost, to Edith D'Addario, director of the Joffrey Ballet School, for her support, encouragement, and contributions to adult ballet education; it was her commitment to the project that made this book possible; to Florence Lessing, one of the first to support and encourage the adult dance student; to Andrei Kulyk, Joffrey School teacher, historian, musician, and friend; to Dorothy Lister, teacher and teacher's teacher; and to Joffrey School faculty members Liz D'Anna, Sidney Lowenthal, Zelma Bustillo, Eleanor D'Antuono, and Trinette Singleton, pianist Paul Spong, and everyone at the Joffrey Ballet School who saw us through this project.

Special thanks to photographer Steve Ladner for seeing, sensing, and capturing the spirit of dance in the Joffrey School, and to Evie Vlahakis, our consulting physical therapist, for her knowledge and assistance in seeing that the workout was not only fun but safe (and who, we're proud to say, became a dedicated adult ballet enthusiast in the process). Thank you, too, to Luc Bouchard and the wonderful make-up artists of M.A.C. Cosmetics for donating their time and expertise to making our beautiful faculty and students even more so.

We also wish to thank the editors at St. Martin's Press; our sensitive copy editor, Bruce Macomber; Geoff Bailey for his tireless efforts on the Source Directory; and John Moss for additional research; Marion Horosko of *Dance* magazine for her ready advice and continuing encouragement; K. C. Patrick, editor of *Dance Theater Now*, and Virginia Spatz, editor of *Dancing Through Life*, for putting us in touch with adult ballet enthusiasts across the country (a special thank you, Virginia, for graciously making the *Ballet-Fit* questionnaire available to your readers); and, of course, thank you to the many adult students at the Joffrey Ballet School and at other schools and studios across the country who took the time to fill out our questionnaires, share their experiences, enthusiasm, and goals, serving as examples and inspiration.

Most of all, our thanks to the Joffrey Ballet School students: to the beautiful and talented advanced students who appear on these pages—Noelle Doner, Felise Bagley, Kiyoko Gotonda, Teanna Zarro, Andres Neira, and Greg Stuart (one and all, another source of inspiration); and especially to all the adult students and faculty who gave of their time and allowed us to photograph them in their classes. Thank you, see you in class!

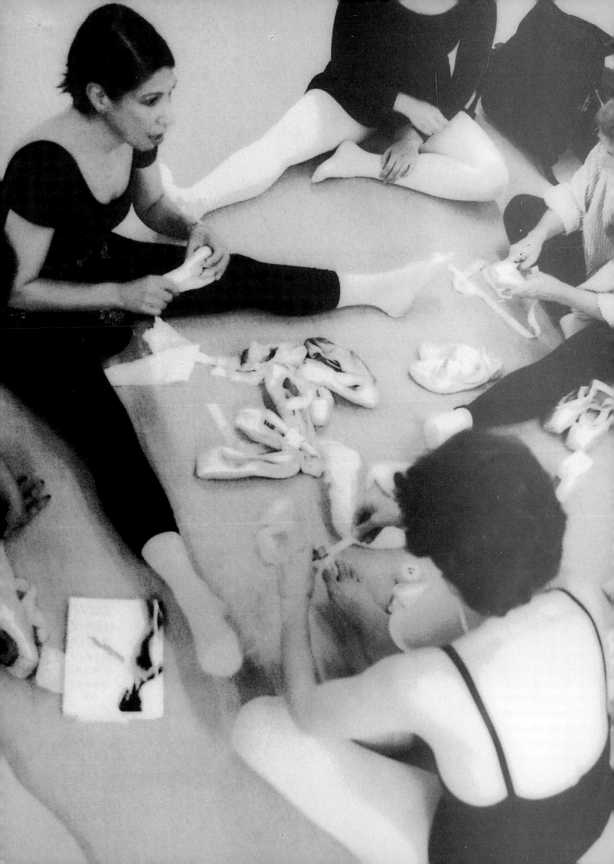

THE BALLET-FIT SOURCE DIRECTORY

The listings below represent a sampling of ballet publications, audio and videotapes, books and CD-ROMs, dancewear and footwear suppliers, schools that have answered our questionnaire and are receptive to adult students, universities with dance education and other programs, and other resources, all of interest to the adult ballet student.

Audio and Video

Asgard Productions
1548 Beechwood Cove
Virginia Beach, VA 23464
(804) 467-4420
A complete mail-order catalog of music for contemporary ballet and modern dance.

The Balanced Body Mat Program
Distributed by Current Concepts Corp.
Call (800) 240-3539 to order.
An 87-minute video of mat exercises and stretches.

Ballet 1
Text by Josephine Holling; music by Kevin Chapman
by Time Tapes, for the Royal Academy of Dancing
Distributed by Professional and Educational Training Aids, Ltd.

127 High Street
Hampton Hill
Middlesex TW12 INJ
  England
Beginner ballet classes on cassette available from Freed's of London.

Ballet CD-ROM
  by Victoria Morgan
Call (800) 600-6568 to order.
Over 700 steps demonstrated. Interactive history of ballet and advice from professional dancers.

Ballet Dynamics, Inc.
163 Amsterdam Avenue
Suite 234
New York, NY 10023
(800) 357-3525
Mail-order catalog with wide selection of videos and CDs.

Beginnings
Box 626

Radio City Station
New York, NY 10101
Call (800) 411-3740 for free catalog.
Ballet-oriented movement-analysis videocassettes.

Hoctor Products
Box 38
Waldwick, NJ 07463
(800) 462-8679
Distributors of dance publications, cassettes, and other media, including those by Lynn Stanford and David Howard.

JAY Distributors
Box 191332
Dallas, TX 75219
(800) 793-6843
Fax: (214) 526-0223
On-line: www.flash.net/~jaydist
Distributors of recordings on cassette and CD for use in dance training.

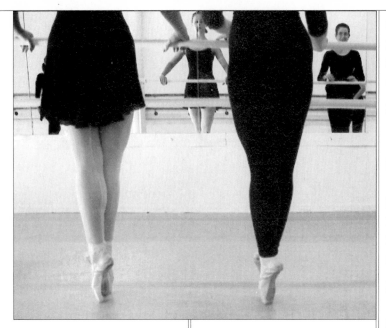

Penguin Books
375 Hudson Street
New York, NY 10014
(212) 366-2000

*Basic Principles of Classical
Ballet: Russian Ballet
Technique*
by Agrippina Vaganova; trans-
lated by Anatole Chujoy
Dover Publishers
180 Varick Street
New York, NY 10013
(212) 255-6399

*Dance Book Club / Princeton
Book Co.*
Box 57
Pennington, NJ 08534
Call (800) 220-7149 for a free
catalog.
On-line:
http://www.dancehorizons.com
*Wide selection of dance books
and videos. Titles include:*
Both Sides of the Mirror
by Anna Paskevska
*First Steps in Ballet: Basic
Exercises at the Barre*
by Thalia Mara
*Second Steps in Ballet: Basic
Center Exercises*
by Thalia Mara
*Third Steps in Ballet: Basic
Allegro Steps*
by Thalia Mara
*Fourth Steps in Ballet: On Your
Toes! Basic Pointe*
by Thalia Mara

Roper Records
45-15 21st Street
Long Island City, NY 11101
Call (718) 786-2401 for a free
catalog.
*Retail-store and mail-order cata-
log of music for ballet training.*

Envision Video
Magazine/Instructional Dance
Videotapes
(800) 800-5437
On-line: http//www.arts-
online.com/Roe.html

Zena Rommett Floor-Barre
Technique
Distributed by Zena Rommett
Dance Association
Call (212) 633-0352 to order.
*Video of basic barre technique.
Available from fine dance stores
or by mail.*

Books

A Dictionary of Ballet Terms
by Leo Kersley and Janet
Sinclair
Da Capo Press
Plenum Publishing
Corporation
233 Spring Street
New York, NY 10013

Ballet: An Illustrated History
by Mary Clarke and Clement
Crisp
Published by Hamish
Hamilton, Ltd.
Available in the United States
from Books Britain
(212) 749-4713
Fax: (212) 749-7509

Basic Ballet: The Steps Defined
by Joyce Mackie

Dance! Therapy for Dancers
  by Beryl Dunn
Photos by Philip Raymond-
  Barker
Published by Heinemann
  Health Books, London
Available in the United States
  from Books Britain
(212) 749-4713
Fax: (212) 749-7509

Inside Ballet Technique
  by Valerie Grieg
Princeton Book Company
Box 57
Pennington, NJ 08534
(800) 200-7149

*Step-by-Step Ballet Class: The
  Official Illustrated Guide*
by the Royal Academy of
  Dancing
Published by Contemporary
  Publishing
4255 West Touhy Avenue
Lincolnwood, IL 60646
(800) 323-4900

*Technical Manual and
  Dictionary of Classical Ballet*
by Gail Grant; illustrated by the
  author
Dover Publications
180 Varick Street
New York, NY
(212) 255-6399

Health and Medical
Advice

The Dancer's Book of Health

by L. M. Vincent, M.D.
Princeton Book Company
Box 57
Pennington, NJ 08534
(800) 220-7149

Diet for Dancers
by Robin D. Chmelar and Sally
  S. Fitt
A Dance Horizons Book
Princeton Book Company
Box 57
Pennington, NJ 08534
(800) 220-7149

Harkness Center for Dance
  Injuries, A Program of the
  Hospital for Joint Diseases
301 East 17th Street
New York, NY 10003
(212) 598-6022
Fax: (212) 598-6249

*Preventing Dance Injuries: An
  Interdisciplinary Perspective*
Edited by Ruth Solomon,
  Sandra C. Minton, and John
  Solomon
Published by American Alliance
  for Health, Physical
  Education, Recreation and
  Dance
1900 Association Drive
Reston, VA 22091
Call (800) 321-0789 to order.

Dancewear

Angelo Luzio Dancewear
Place Picasso
Montreal, Canada
H1P 3J8
(514) 322-8350
*Makers of dancewear. Available
  from retail dance stores in
  Canada and the United States.*

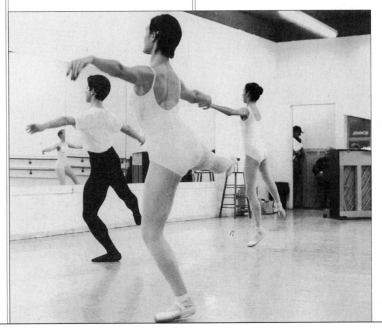

Back Bay Dancewear
181 Massachusetts Avenue
Boston, MA 02115
(800) 554-2340
Complete discount mail-order catalog, carrying Freed, Angelo Luzio, Capezio, and other top-quality products.

Ballet Etc.
Call (800) DANCE-25.
Mail-order catalog with full selection of shoes and dancewear.

Bareca Dancewear
Call 888-BALLET-1 for a free catalog.

Baryshnikov Dance Collection Dancewear
8960 Carroll Way
San Diego, CA 92121

(800) 666-2127
Footwear
22-60 46th Street
Long Island City, NY 11105
(800) 272-6033
Makers of footwear and dancewear available at fine dance retailers.

Body Wrappers
1350 Broadway
New York, NY 10018
(212) 279-3492
Dancewear available from retail stores and mail-order catalogs nationwide.

Capezio
One Campus Road
Totowa, NJ 07512
(800) 234-4858
On-line: http://www.capezio.com

Quality dancewear and accessories available through Capezio retail stores nationwide.

Cathy Hazeltine
501 Gleasondale Road
Stowe, MA 01775
Call (800) 270-9111 for a free catalog.
Dancewear available in fine retail stores or by mail.

Dance Distributors
Box 11440
Harrisburg, PA 17108
Call (800) 33-DANCE for free catalog.
Complete discount catalog, including such brands as Capezio, Baryshnikov, Danskin, and Freed's of London.

The Dance Shop
2485 Forest Park Blvd.
Fort Worth, TX 76110
Call (800) 22-DANCE for a free catalog.
Top name brands available by mail from their store in Fort Worth.

Dansant Boutique
6623 Old Dominion Drive
McLean, VA 22101
(800) DAN-SANT
On-line: http://www.dansant.com/ftp.dansant.com

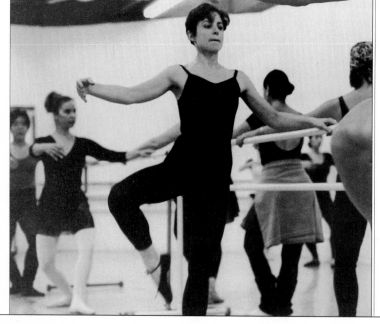

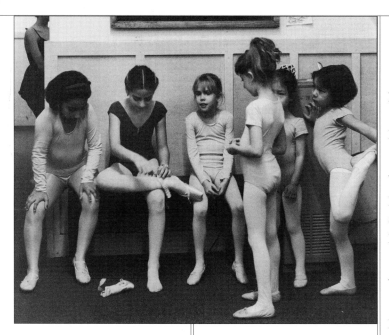

Discount Dance Supply
Call (800) 328-7107 for a free
    catalog.
On-line:
    http://www.discdance.com
*Dancewear at discount prices.
    Brand names include Grishko,
    Danskin, Bodywrappers,
    Baryshnikov, and more.*

Freed's of London
922 Seventh Avenue
New York, NY
(800) 835-1701
*Available by mail through their
    retail store in New York or from
    fine dancewear stores across the
    country.*

Grishko
1655 Mt. Pleasant Rd.
Villanova, PA 19085
(610) 527-9553

*Makers of high quality pointe
    shoes. Available at fine retail
    stores.*

Harmonie
3131 Western Avenue, Suite 327
Seattle, WA 98121
(800) 435-4518
*Dance knitwear available from
    quality retail stores.*

Illinois Theatrical
Box 34284
Chicago, IL 60634
(800) 745-3777
*Offering a wide selection of
    wholesale dancewear and
    shoes. Shipping is free for
    orders over $100.*

Lynch's
939 Howard
Dearborn, MI 48124

(800) 24-LYNCH
*Wide selection of dancewear and
    shoes available by mail.*

New York Dancewear Company
188-06 Union Turnpike
Flushing, NY 11366
(800) 755-DANCE
Discount dancewear catalog.

Prima Soft
842 Red Lion Road
Philadelphia, PA 19115
(215) 676-5777
*Dancewear and dance accessories
    available from fine retail stores.*

Russian Class
3253 Braza Drive, #2
Ann Arbor, MI 48018
888-4RCLASS
*Handmade ballet shoes available
    for custom order.*

Sansha USA
1733 Broadway
New York, NY 10019
(800) 392-5246
*High-quality ballet shoes avail-
    able by mail from manufactur-
    ers and from fine retail stores
    across the country.*

Southern Dance Supply
7125 Capitol Boulevard
Raleigh, NC 27616
Call (800) 872-0883 for a free
    catalog.
*Save 25 percent or more on
    Capezio, Bloch, Sansha,
    Grishko and more.*

Star Styled Dance and
   Bodywear
Box 119029
Hialeah, FL 33011
(800) 5-DANCER
*Dancewear and accessories avail-
   able for mail order.*

Victoria's
1331 Lincoln Avenue
San Jose, CA 95125
(800) 626-9258
*Discount prices on dancewear,
   barres, mirrors, mats and
   more. All available by mail.*

Equipment

Alva's Ballet Barres
1417 West 8th Street
San Pedro, CA 90732
(310) 519-1314
Barres available by mail.

Ballet Barres
Box 261206
Tampa, FL 33685
*For a free catalog of barres, call
   800-767-1199.*

Eurotard
1328 Union Hill Road
Alpharetta, GA 30201
(770) 475-3045
Makers of pointe *shoe pads.
   Available at fine dancewear
   stores.*

Panache International, Inc.
Box 5332
Chesapeake, VA 23324

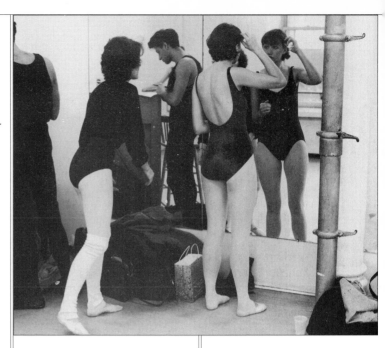

888-66-DANCE
*Makers of portable ballet barres.
   Available at many retail stores
   or can be ordered by mail.*

Publications

Ballet Is Fun
Call 800-678-8014, ext. 700, to
   order.

*Dance and the Arts: Life and
   International Travel*
Published by Dance Pages, Inc.
200 West 72nd Street
New York, NY 10023
(800) 584-5428

Dance Magazine
33 West 60th Street
New York, NY 10023
(800) 331-1750
Monthly magazine with features

*on leading dance personalities,
news, and reviews, "The Young
Dancer" and other items of
interest to dance students and
teachers.*
On-line: http://www.
dancemagazine.com

Dance Teacher Now
P. O. Box 41204
Raleigh, NC 27629-1204
(800) 362-6765
On-line: http://www.dance-
teacher.com
*Bimonthly magazine with com-
plete list of back articles from
1979 to the present. Articles
can be requested for a charge of
$2.00.*

Dancing Through Life
Box 15087

Washington, DC 20003-0087
(202) 543-4921
E-mail: vspatz@access.digex.net
Bimonthly publication by and for adult students of dance and their teachers. Free samples to readers of Ballet-Fit *upon request.*

Schools & Universities

Regional Dance America
  Association
c/o Allegro Ballet
1570 South Derry Ashford
Suite 100
Houston, TX 77077

(713) 496-4670
National Association of Schools
  of Dance (NASD)
11250 Roger Bacon Drive,
  Suite 21
Reston, VA 20190
(703) 437-0700

Alabama

Exclusively Dance
7154 Cahaba Valley Road
Birmingham, AL 35203
(205) 995-9220

Alabama Dance Theatre
1018 Madison Avenue
Montgomery, AL 36104

(334) 241-2590
Huntingdon College
Performing Arts-Dance
  Program
1500 East Fairview Avenue
Montgomery, AL 36106-2148
(334) 833-4538
Fax: (334) 833-4486

Arizona

Arizona State University
Department of Dance
Box 870304
Tempe, AZ 85287-0304
(602) 965-5029
Fax: (602) 965-2247
Choreography

Arkansas

Arkansas Ballet Academy
Box 7574
Little Rock, AR 72217
(501) 664-9509

California

Scripps College
Dance Department
1030 Columbia Avenue
Claremont, CA 91711
(909) 607-2934
Fax: (909) 621-8323
Dance major or minor

Orange Coast College
Dance Department
2701 Fairview Road
Box 5005
Costa Mesa, CA 92628-5005

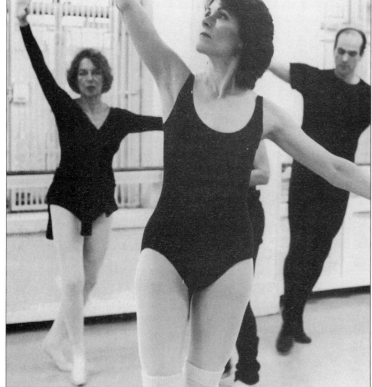

(714) 432-5506
Fax: (714) 432-5934

California State University-
  Hayward
Theatre and Dance Department
25800 Carlos Bee Boulevard
Hayward, CA 94542
(510) 885-3118
Fax: (510) 885-4748

Mills College
Dance Department
5000 MacArthur Boulevard
Oakland, CA 94613
(510) 430-2175
Fax: (510) 430-3314
Modern dance, choreography,
  history, theory, and technique

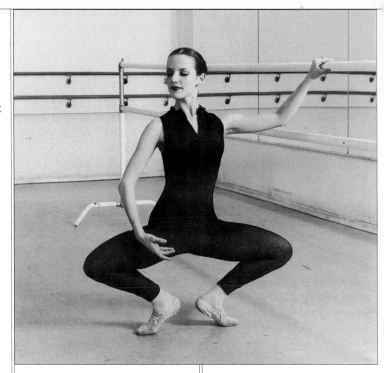

The Academy of Ballet
2121 Market Street
San Francisco, CA 94114
(415) 552-1166

Ballet Russe
1946 Clement Street
San Francisco, CA 94121
(415) 386-3560

Brady Street Dance Center
60 Brady Street
San Francisco, CA 94103
(415) 558-9355

City Ballet School
44 Page Street
San Francisco, CA 94102
(415) 626-8878

Duets Dance Studio
4504 Irving Street

San Francisco, CA 94122
(415) 665-5712

San Francisco Dance Center
Home of Lines Contemporary
  Ballet
50 Oak Street, 4th Floor
San Francisco, CA 94102
(415) 863-3229

Meredith Baylis' American
  Dance Institute
12745 Ventura Boulevard
Studio City, CA 91604
(818) 760-2167

Colorado

Aspen Ballet Company and
  School
750 Meadowwood Drive

Aspen, CO 81611
(970) 925-7175

Absolute Beginners—Adult
  Ballet
Denver, CO 80203
(303) 839-5992

Academy of Colorado Ballet
1278 Lincoln Street
Denver, CO 80203
(303) 837-8888

The Ballet School
2385 South Downing Street
Denver, CO 80210
(303) 698-1739
Choreography, Laban movement
  analysis, and historic dance
  forms

University of Northern
  Colorado
Theatre and Dance Department
Dance Program
Frasier 108
Greeley, CO 80639
(970) 351-2597
Fax: (970) 351-1923
*Teaching/movement analysis,
  dance sciences, theatre arts
  with emphasis on dance*

Connecticut

D'Valda and Sirico's Dance
  Center
1580 Post Road
Fairfield, CT 06430
(203) 255-9440

Hartford Conservatory
Diploma School
834 Asylum Avenue
Hartford, CT 06105
(860) 246-2488
Fax: (860) 249-6330
Diploma in dance pedagogy

School of the Hartford Ballet
224 Farmington Avenue
Hartford, CT 06105-3501
(860) 525-9396
Fax: (860) 249-8116
*Adult evening classes during the
  academic year and throughout
  the summer. National
  Association of Schools of Dance
  (NASD) accredited institution.*

Connecticut Ballet Center

20 Acosta Street
Stamford, CT 06902
(203) 978-0771

Connecticut College
New London, CT 06320-4196
(860) 439-2830
*BA in dance/choreography and
  dance studies.*

District of Columbia

Academy of Theatrical Arts
1747 Connecticut Avenue, NW
Washington, DC 20004
(202) 462-2266

American University
Performing Arts
4400 Massachusetts Ave., NW
Washington, DC 20016
(202) 885-3424

Fax: (202) 885-1092
*Musical theatre, interdiscipli-
  nary, dance B.A., M.A.*

St. Mark's Dance Studio
3rd and A Streets, S.E.
Washington, DC 20003
(202) 543-0054

Taps and Company
410 8th Street, N.W. #210
Washington, DC 20004
(202) 393-TAPS

Washington School of Ballet
3515 Wisconsin Avenue, N.W.
Washington, DC 20016
(202) 362-1683

Florida

Aventura Dance Academy
19048 N.E. 29th Avenue
Aventura, FL 33180
(305) 935-3232

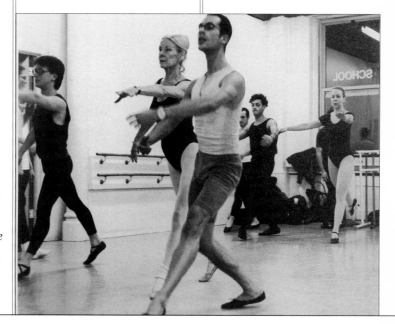

Ballet Academy of Miami
1809 Ponce de Leon Boulevard
Coral Gables, FL 33134
(305) 444-3331

Dance Dimensions
5303–5307 North Dixie
  Highway
Fort Lauderdale, FL 33334
(305) 491-4668

Florida State University
404 Montgomery Gym
Tallahassee, FL 32306
(904) 644-1023
NASD accredited institution.

Florida Dance Conservatory
3915 Havervill Road, North
West Palm Beach, FL 33417
(407) 478-7722

Georgia

University of Georgia

Department of Dance
Sanford Drive
Athens, GA 30602-3653
(706) 542-4415
Fax: (706) 542-4084
*Pre-dance therapy, studio man-
  agement, teacher certification*

Atlanta School of Ballet
4279 Roswell Road, Suite 703
Atlanta, GA 30342
(404) 303-1501

Price Performing Arts Center
5495 Old National Highway
Atlanta, GA 30349
(404) 305-8812

The Studio—Atlanta Dance
3229 Cains Hill Place, N.W.
Atlanta, GA 30305
(404) 233-8686

Brenau University
Arts and Sciences

One Centennial Circle
Gainesville, GA 30501
(770) 534-6249
Fax: (770) 534-6114
*Dance pedagogy, dance perfor-
mance, arts management*

Hawaii

University of Hawaii-Manoa
Department of Theatre and
  Dance
1770 East West Road
Honolulu, HI 96822
(808) 956-7622
Fax: (808) 956-4234
*Dance ethnology, several forms of
  Asian-Pacific dance*

Academy of Dance Spectrum
  Hawaii
Kailua, HI 96734
(808) 254-3116

Idaho

Ballet Idaho Academy of Dance
501 South 8th Street
Boise, ID 83702
(208) 336-3241

University of Idaho
Center for Dance, Division of
  HPERD
Moscow, ID 83844-2401
(208) 885-7921
Fax: (208) 885-5929
*Dance education, dance peda-
  gogy*

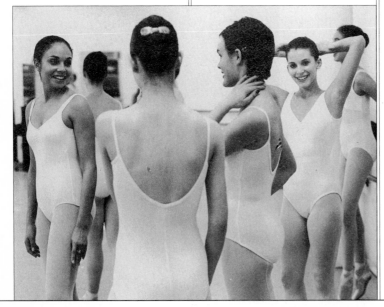

Illinois

Beverly Art Center Dance
  Studio
2324 West 111th
Chicago, IL 60643
(773) 445-3838

Chicago Multi-Cultural Dance
  Center
Home of Bryant Ballet
806 South Plymouth Court
Chicago, IL 60605
(312) 461-0030

Columbia College
Dance Department
4730 North Sheridan Road
Chicago, IL 60640
(773) 989-3310
Fax: (773) 271-7046
Teaching

Conservatory of Dance
10339 South Pulaski Road
Chicago, IL 60655
(773) 239-2042

Darla's Dance Center
6236 South Central
Chicago, IL 60638
(773) 581-1350

Joel Hall Dance Center
934 West North Avenue
Chicago, IL 60622
(312) 587-1122

Lou Conte Dance Studios
218 South Wabash Avenue
Chicago, IL 60604
(312) 461-0892

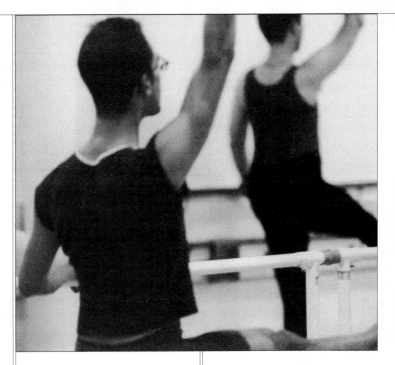

Ruth Page Foundation School
  of Dance
1016 North Dearborn Street
Chicago, IL 60610
(312) 337-6543

Northwestern University
Dance Program in the Theatre
1979 South Campus Drive
Evanston, IL 60208-2430
(847) 491-3147
Fax: (847) 467-2019
*Master of arts in theater/dance
  emphasis*

University of Illinois, Urbana-
  Champaign
Department of Dance
907½ West Nevada
Urbana, IL 61801-3810
(217) 333-1010

Fax: (217) 333-3000
*Undergraduate and graduate;
  NASD accredited institution.*

Kansas

University of Kansas
Music and Dance
452 Murphy Hall
Lawrence, KS 66045
(913) 864-4264
Fax: (913) 864-5387

American Dance Center
11728 Quivira Road
Overland Park, KS 66210
(913) 451-3020

Maryland

Ballet Theatre of Annapolis
  School

Maryland Hall
801 Chase Street
Annapolis, MD 21401
(410) 263-8289

Ballet Academy of Baltimore
1500 Serpentine Road
Baltimore, MD 21209
(410) 337-7974

Goucher College
Dance Department
1021 Dulaney Valley Road
Baltimore, MD 21204
(410) 337-6390
Fax: (410) 337-6123
Dance education, dance history, performance and choreography, arts administration, dance and theatre, dance therapy, and dance science

Academy of the Maryland
    Youth Ballet
7702 Woodmont Avenue, #203
Bethesda, MD 20814
(301) 652-2232

Dawn Crafton Dance Centre
7601 C Airpark Road
Gaithersburg, MD 20879
(301) 840-8400

Massachusetts

Hampshire College
School of Humanities and
    Arts—Dance Program
Dance Building
Amherst, MA 01002
(413) 582-5674

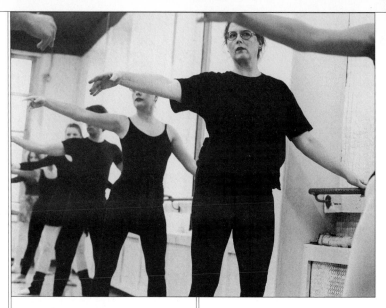

Fax: (413) 582-5481
Pre-dance therapy

Ballet Theatre of Boston
186 Massachusetts Avenue
Boston, MA 02115
(617) 262-0961

Boston Ballet Company
19 Clarendon Street
Boston, MA 02116
(617) 695-6950

Michigan

Birmingham Ballet and Jazz
    School
The Community House
380 South Bates Street
Birmingham, MI 48009
(248) 644-5832

Wayne State University
Dance Department
125 Matthaei Building

Detroit, MI 48202
(313) 577-4273
Fax: (313) 577-5691
Ballet, choreography / education, B.S. in dance, teacher certification, K–12

Hope College
Dow Center
Box 9000
Holland, MI 49422
(616) 395-7700
Dance performance/choreography, dance psychology, dance education, dance theater, dance administration, dance medicine, dance engineering; NASD accredited institution.

Western Michigan University
Dalton Center
Kalamazoo, MI 49008
(616) 387-1000
NASD accredited institution.

Academy of Dance Arts
2224 East Michigan
Lansing, MI 48912
(517) 372-9887

Minnesota

Minnesota Ballet
506 West Michigan Street
Duluth, MN 55802
(218) 733-7570

Ballet Arts Minnesota
528 Hennepin Avenue, #201
Minneapolis, MN 55403
(612) 340-1071

Zenon Dance Company and
  School
528 Hennepin #400
Minneapolis, MN 55403
(612) 338-1101

Saint Olaf College
1520 Saint Olaf Avenue
Northfield, MN 55057
(507) 646-2222

Mississippi

University of Southern
  Mississippi
Southern Station
Box 5052
Hattiesburg, MS 39406
NASD accredited institution.

Tupelo Academy of Dance Arts
1016 24th Avenue
Meridian, MS 39301
(601) 693-2331

Missouri

School of the Westport Ballet
3936 Main Street
Kansas City, MO 64111
(816) 531-4330

Ballet Center of St. Louis
10 Kimler Drive
St. Louis, MO 63043
(314) 991-1233

Washington University
Performing Arts
W.U. Campus Box 1108
1 Brookings Drive
St. Louis, MO 63143
(314) 935-5858
Fax: (314) 935-4955
Dance emphasis major

New Hampshire

Antioch New England Graduate
  School
40 Avon Street
Keene, NH 03431
(603) 257-3122
M.A. in dance/movement
  therapy; minor in counseling
  psychology; and an M.Ed. in
  dance/movement therapy

Granite State Ballet School
36 Arlington Street
Nashua, NH 03060
(603) 889-8408

School of New England Ballet
Box 4501
135 Daniels Street

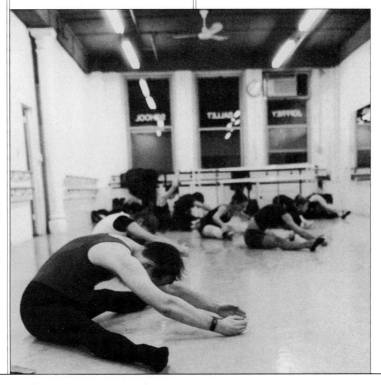

Portsmouth, NH 03802
(603) 430-9309

New Jersey

Dancing Arts Center
One Pleasant Street
Hackensack, NJ 01701
(508) 875-0931

Dinshah Dance Studio
Delsea Drive
Malaga, NJ 08328
(609) 694-3555

Rutgers University
Box 270
Marryott Music Building
New Brunswick, NJ 08903
(732) 932-1766
NASD accredited institution.

Royal Academy of Dancing
17 Franklin Place
Rutherford, NJ 07070
(201) 438-4400
Fax: (201) 438-4552
Dance teacher training; correspondence courses in dance history, anatomy, ballet, child psychology and development; music teaching certificate, teaching diploma, advanced teaching diploma

Montclair State University
Dept. of Theater and Dance
Life Hall
Upper Montclair, NJ 07043
(201) 655-4217
Fax: (201) 655-5279

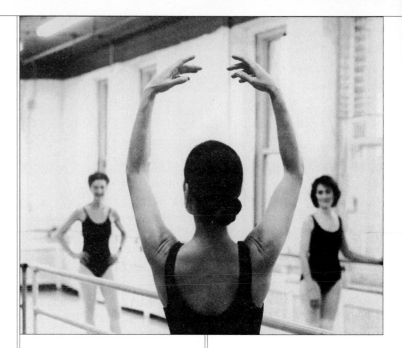

Courses in ballet, choreography, history; NASD accredited institution.

New Mexico

Ballet Theatre of New Mexico
6913 Natalie N.E.
Albuquerque, MN 87110
(505) 888-1054

Dance Theatre of the Southwest
4200 Wyoming Northeast
Albuquerque, NM
(505) 296-9465

University of New Mexico
Albuquerque, NM 87131
(505) 277-3660
B.A. and M.A.; Department of Theatre and Dance

New York

Studios in New York are far too numerous to list in full. The listing below is just a sampling of what is available.

State University of New York—
Brockport
Dance Department
350 New Campus Drive
Brockport, NY 14420-2939
(716) 395-2153
Fax: (716) 395-5134
Choreography, education, dance science and somantics; NYS K–12 certification; NASD accredited institution.

State University of New York—
Buffalo
Department of Theatre and Dance

285 Alumni Arena
Buffalo, NY 14260-6030
(716) 645-6898
Fax: (716) 645-6992
Music theatre, preparation for teaching, choreography, health- and recreation-related research

State University of New York–Geneseo
School of Performing Arts
1 College Circle
Geneseo, NY 14454
(716) 245-5824
Fax: (716) 245-5826
Minor in dance; concentration in dance

Ballet Academy East
1651 Third Avenue
New York, NY 10128
(212) 410-9140

Barnard College
3009 Broadway
New York, NY 10027
(212) 854-5262
NASD accredited school.

Carol Rioux Ballet New York
237 West 54th Street
New York, NY 10019
(212) 631-1013
Mailing address:
c/o Barbara Marcel
213 Cornwall Road
Glen Rock, NJ 07452

Joffrey Ballet School
434 Avenue of the Americas
New York, NY 10011
(212) 254-8520
NASD accredited institution.

New York Theatre Ballet School
30 East 31st Street, 5th Floor

New York, NY 10016
(212) 679-0401

New York University
35 West 4th Street, Suite 675
New York, NY 10012
(212) 998-5400
Dance in higher education; dance K–12; NASD accredited institution.

Merce Cunningham Studio
55 Bethune Street
New York, NY 10014
(212) 255-3130
NASD accredited institution.

Steps Studio
2121 Broadway
New York, NY 10023
(212) 874-2410

Teachers College
Columbia University
Dance and Dance Education Program
Box 139
New York, NY 10027
(212) 678-3328
Fax: (212) 678-4048
Dance and dance education

Central Park Dance Studio
450 Central Park Avenue
Scarsdale, NY 10583
(914) 723-2940

North Carolina

Charlotte City Ballet School
8612 Monroe Road
Charlotte, NC 28212

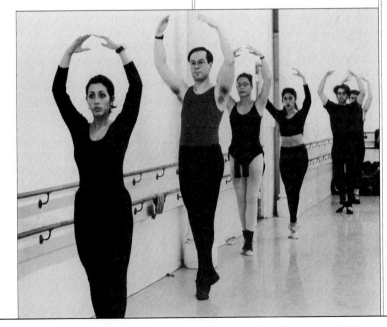

(704) 536-0615

University of North Carolina—
  Charlotte
Department of Dance and
  Theatre
9201 University City Boulevard
Charlotte, NC 28223-0001
(704) 547-2482
Fax: (704) 547-3795
Dance, dance education, theatre,
  theatre education

The School of Greensboro
  Ballet
200 North Davie Street
Greensboro, NC 27401
(910) 333-7480

Raleigh School of Ballet
3921 Beryl Road
Raleigh, NC 27401
(919) 834-9261

Catawba College
Theatre Arts
2300 West Innes Street
Salisbury, NC 28144
  800/CATAWBA
Fax: (704) 637-4444
Minor in dance; major and minor
  in musical theatre or theatre
  arts; major in theatre arts
  administration; minor in studio
  art

Ohio

University of Akron
School of Dance
354 East Market Street

Akron, OH 44325-2502
(330) 972-7948
Musical theatre/dance, K–12 cer-
  tification; NASD accredited
  institution.

Ohio University
Rufus Putnam Hall 222
Athens, OH 45701
(614) 593-1000
NASD accredited institution.

Ann Fine Ballet Center
5208 Beechmont Avenue
Cincinnati, OH 45230
(513) 231-3580

University of Cincinnati
Conservatory of Music
Box 210003
Cincinnati, OH 45221
(513) 556-2700
NASD accredited institution.

Ohio State University
1813 North High Street
Columbus, OH 43210
(614) 292-7977
Fax: (614) 292-0939
Dance performance, dance edu-
  cation, notation, production;
  NASD accredited institution.

Oregon

The Conservatory of Classical
  Dance
456 Charnelton
Eugene, OR 97401
(541) 345-3632

University of Oregon
Department of Dance
1214 University of Oregon
Eugene, OR 97403-1214
(541) 346-3386
Undergraduate major and minor

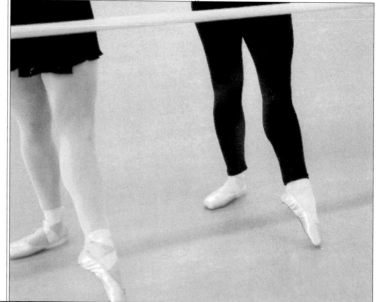

in dance; graduate emphasis in
choreography, dance history,
ethnology or dance science

Mainstreet Dance Studio
231 East Main Street
Hillsboro, OR 97123
(503) 693-6166

Pennsylvania

Muhlenberg College
Department of Theater Arts
Baker Center for the Arts
2400 Chew Street
Allentown, PA 18104
(610) 821-3335
Fax: (610) 821-3633
Dance major or minor; theatre
arts major

Broadway Dance Academy
258 Main Street
East Greenville, PA 18041
(215) 679-4488

Mercyhurst College
Dance Department
501 East 38th Street
Erie, PA 16546
(814) 824-2587
Fax: (814) 824-2055
Performance and teaching/chore-
ography concentrations; dance,
arts administration; dance
movement/art therapy minors;
returning professor program

The Rock School of
  Pennsylvania Ballet
1101 South Broad Street

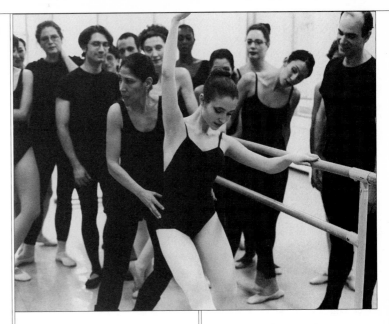

Philadelphia, PA 19147
(215) 551-7010
Fax: (215) 551-8538

Rhode Island

Brae Crest School of Ballet
Sherman
Lincoln, RI 02865
(401) 334-2560

South Carolina

Columbia College
1301 Columbia College Drive
Columbia, SC 29203
(803) 786-3847
B.A. in dance education; NASD
accredited institution.

Tennessee

Columbia State Community
  College

Commercial Entertainment
104 Yates Drive
Franklin, TN 37064
(615) 790-4420
Dance studio management

Ballet Memphis
Box 11136
Memphis, TN 38111
(901) 763-0139

Nashville Ballet
2976 Sidco Drive
Nashville, TN 37204
(615) 244-7233

Texas

Texas Woman's University
Programs in Dance
Box 425708
Denton, TX 76204-5619
(817) 898-2085
Fax: (817) 898-2098

Choreography, teaching, research

Allegro Ballet
1570 South Derry Ashford
Suite 100
Houston, TX 77077
(713) 496-4670

Allen Darnel Beginners—Only
    Adult Dance Studio
5959 Westheimer Road
Houston, TX 77057
(713) 789-3262

American Academy of Dance
15775 Bammel Village Drive
Houston, TX 77014
(281) 444-9698

City Dance Studio
5925 Kirby Avenue
Houston, TX 77075
(713) 529-6100

Houston Academy of Ballet
14520 Memorial Drive, Suite 78
Houston, TX 77079
(281) 497-4783

Houston Ballet Academy
Box 130487
1921 West Bell
Houston, TX 77219-0487
(713) 523-6300
NASD accredited institution.

Houston Metropolitan Dance
    Center
1202 Calumet Street
Houston, TX 77004
(713) 522-6375

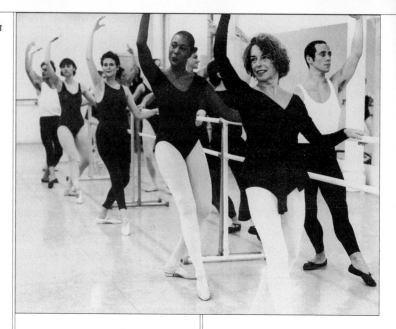

Utah

University of Utah
Department of Ballet
110 Mariott Center for Dance
Salt Lake City, UT 84112
(801) 581-8231
Fax: (801) 581-5442
Ballet, teaching

Virginia

Arlington Center for Dance
3808 Wilson Boulevard
Arlington, VA 22203
(703) 522-2414

Ravel Studio of Ballet and Jazz
10130 Colvin Run Road
Great Falls, VA 22066
(703) 759-1516

Studio of Classical Ballet
Box 46

Great Falls, VA 22066
(703) 759-3366

Shenandoah University
Dance Division
1460 University Drive
Winchester, VA 22601-5195
(540) 665-4565
Fax: (540) 665-5402
Dance education

Washington

Nancy Whyte School of Ballet
Box 2393
Bellingham, WA 98227
(360) 734-9141

Cornish College of the Arts
Dance Department
710 East Roy
Seattle, WA 98102
(800) 726-ARTS

Fax: (206) 720-1011
Teaching

Dance Theatre Northwest
6908 West 27th Street
University Place, WA 98466
(206) 565-5149

Pacific Northwest Ballet School
301 Mercer Street
Seattle, WA 98109
(206) 441-2435

Jo Emery Ballet School
2315 Sixth Avenue
Tacoma, WA 98403
(206) 759-5714

Wisconsin

Green Bay School of Dance
129 South Washington Street
Green Bay, WI 54301
(414) 433-9510

University of Wisconsin—
   Madison
Dance Department
139 Lathrop Hall
1050 University Avenue
Madison, WI 53706
(608) 262-1691
Fax: (608) 265-3841
Education, interarts, and tech-
   nology

Milwaukee Ballet School
504 West National Avenue
Milwaukee, WI 53204
(414) 649-4077

University of Wisconsin—

Stevens Point
Fine Arts Center
Stevens Point, WI 54481
(715) 346-0123
NASD accredited institution.

Central Wisconsin School of
   Ballet
124 North Third Avenue
Wausau, WI 54401
(715) 842-4447

Canada

National Ballet School
105 Maitland Street
Toronto, Ontario
M6G 1Y1
CANADA
(416) 964-3780
Fax: (416) 964-5135
Professional ballet/academic,
   grades 5 to 12; teacher training
   1 to 3 years, summer teachers'
   seminar

Royal Academy of Dancing
#404-3284 Yonge Street
Toronto, Ontario
M4N 2L6
CANADA
(416) 489-2813
Fax: (416) 486-3222
Dance teacher training; corre-
   spondence courses in dance his-
   tory, anatomy and ballet/child
   psychology and
   development/music, teaching
   certificate/teaching
   diploma/advanced teaching
   diploma

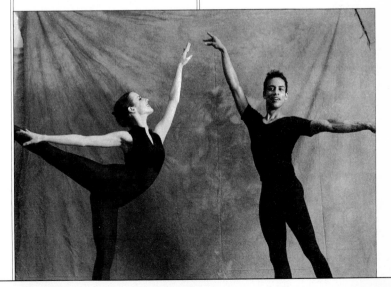

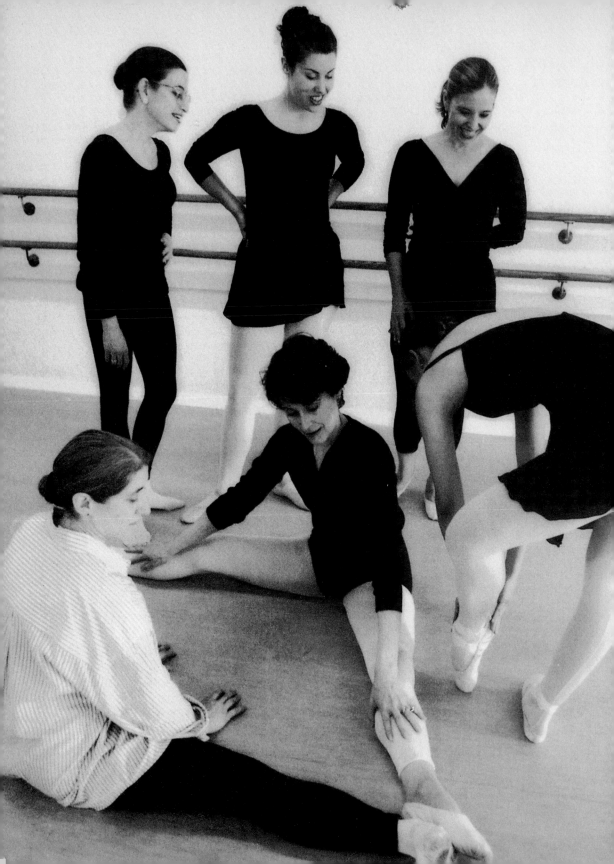

INDEX

A

à la seconde (as a ballet term), 84
abdominal exercises as *Ballet-Fit*
  warm-ups, 155–56, 156
ability, lack of, 18
adagio
  and the *Ballet-Fit* workout,
    176–78
  as a ballet term, 84
  at the barre, 9, 132
  center exercise and, 10
  développés & fondus, 9, 135
advanced class, comparisons with,
  222–23
aerobic workouts, 2–3
affectations, 107–9
Alabama, schools and universities,
  239
alignment, 98
allegro (as a ballet term), 84
ankle weights, 48
appearance (for class)
  hair style, 76–77
  jewelry, makeup and perfume, 77
arabesque, 117
arqué (bow-legged), 44
Arizona, schools and universities,
  239
Arkansas, schools and universities,
  239
arms, use of, 104–5
Arpino, Gerald, 12
attitude, 135
  as a ballet term, 85
  as a social posture. *See* mystique
audio resources, 233–34

B

back problems, 55
  ballet back, 56
  cambré and, 55
  See also foot problems; knee
    problems
balancé, 140
balance, ballet and, 51–52
Balanchine, George, 13
ballet
  other dance forms as comple-
    ments to, 227
ballet back, 56
ballet body, 41–44
  arqué (bow-legged), 44
  hyperextended, 44
  impossible ideal, getting past,
    44–45
  jarreté (knock-kneed), 44
  reshaping, 45–47
  too much too soon, 56–57
  See also physical problems
ballet class
  adult class, 28–29
  asking questions, 32
  ballet as a performing art, 26–28
  "beginners" class, 23–25
  choosing a teacher, 25–26, 30
  favorite spots at the barre, 81–82
  finding, 22–23
  first class, 79–81
  learning with mind and body,
    29–32
  making harder, 110
  more than a workout, 4–7
  professional class, 28–29
  questions to ask, 22–25
  See also terms
ballet class (adult class)
  infantilizing, 28–29
  progress, 35–38
ballet class (typical), 9–10, 39
  at the barre, 9, 39
  in the center, 10, 39
  on the floor, 9–10, 39
Ballet-Fit Source Directory, 233–51
  audio and video, 233–34
  books, 234–35
  dancewear, 235–38
  equipment, 238
  health and medical advice, 235
  publications, 238–239
  schools and universities, 239–51
Ballet-Fit workout (at the barre),
  161–80
  adagio, 176–78
  battements tendus jetés, 170–71
  cambrés, 164–66
  demi-pliés, 162–63
  frappés, 174–75
  grands battements, 179–78
  ronds des jambes, 172–73
  tendus, 167–68
  tendus (optional), 168–69
Ballet-Fit workout (beginning),
  145–49
  bearing arms, 149
  before beginning, 148
  starting position, 148
Ballet-Fit workout (FloorPlay),
  181–95
  buttocks stretch, 194–95

counting music, 110–11
coupés, 134
croisé (as a ballet term), 86

D

dance, pursuing as career, 226
dance bags, 68–69
Dancer's Body Book, The (Kent), 3
dancewear sources, 235–38
D'Anna, Elizabeth, 30–31, 34, 99
dégagés, 9
demi-pliés, 120–22, 138–39
   and the *Ballet-Fit* warm-up, 152
   and the *Ballet-Fit* workout,
     162–63
développés, 9
Diaghilev, Sergei, 13
District of Columbia, schools and
   universities, 241
double leg lifts
   as *Ballet-Fit* FloorPlay, 184–86

E

early training, differences with,
   218–19
Elssler, Fanny, 12
embarrassment, 20
en bas (as a ballet term), 86
en dedans/en dehors (as ballet
   terms), 88
en haut, 125
en l'air (as a ballet term), 88
en point (as a ballet term), 88
endurance, ballet and, 48–49
entrechat sixes
   as *Ballet-Fit* FloorPlay, 190–91
épaulement (as a ballet term), 88
equipment sources, 238
etiquette, 93–97
exercise (ballet), 47–52
   balance, 51–52
   coordination, 52
   endurance, 48–49
   flexibility, 49–51
   for the rest of your life, 58–59

strength, 47–48
expense of ballet class, 19–20
ex-student returning to class, 228
extension (as a ballet term), 87

F

fears (getting past them)
   ability, lack of, 18
   ballet French, 21
   the ballet "look," 20
   class, availability of, 20
   concentration, 21
   coordination, 18–19
   embarrassment, 20
   expense of, 19–20
   feeling out of place, 16–17
   the "girlie-girl" thing, 21
   gracefulness, doubts of, 19
   musicality, lack of, 19
   physical problems, 21–22
   weight worries, 18
feeling out of place, 16–17
fifth position, 102
"find your center" (as a ballet
   term), 89
first position, 100
five positions, 100–103
flamenco
   as complement to ballet, 227
flexibility, ballet and, 49–51
floor exercises (at home), 48
   ankle weights, 48
floor exercises (ballet class), 9–10,
   39
   Ballet-Fit FloorPlay, 181–95
FloorPlay (*Ballet-Fit* workout),
   181–95
   buttocks stretch, 194–95
   double leg lifts, 184–86
   entrechat sixes, 190–91
   hip flexor stretch, 193
   push-ups (men only), 192
   push-ups (modified of women),
     193
   rond de jambe en l'air, 188–89

second position stretches, 182–83
sit-ups, 186–87
Florida, schools and universities,
   241–42
Fokine, Michel, 13
fondu, 9, 134
   as a ballet term, 83
foot problems, 54–55
   ballet feet, 56
   See also back problems; knee
     problems
fourth position, 102
frappés, 9, 130–31
   and the *Ballet-Fit* workout,
     174–75
French
   ballet French, 21, 83
   as the language of ballet, 11, 83

G

Georgia, schools and universities,
   242
"girlie-girl" thing, 21
Giselle, 12, 76
gracefulness, doubts of, 19
grand allegro (center exercise), 10
grands battements, 9, 10, 136
   and the *Ballet-Fit* workout,
     179–80
grands pliés, 120–22
Grant, Gail, 44

H

hair style (for class), 76–77
hamstring stretches
   as *Ballet-Fit* warm-ups, 158
hand movements, 107
Hawaii, schools and universities,
   242
health advice resources, 235
Health magazine, 2, 2–3
hip flexor stretches
   as *Ballet-Fit* FloorPlay, 193
history of ballet, 11–13, 27
   evolution, 11

strength, ballet and, 47–48
stretches
    as *Ballet-Fit* warm-ups, 152, 153
    hamstring stretches, 158
    quadriceps stretches, 159
supporting leg/working leg, 92
surgery, informing teacher of, 221
sweatpants and sweatshirts, 69–70
Sylphide, La, 12, 76

T

Taglioni, Maria, 12
Tai Chi, 2
tap
    as complement to ballet, 227
teachers
    assessing method, 33–34
    choosing, 25–26, 30
    personality problems with, 220-
Technical Manual and Dictionary of
    Classical Ballet (Grant), 44
temps de flèche (as a ballet term), 83
temps lié (as a ballet term), 83
tendus, 9, 123
    as *Ballet-Fit* warm-ups, 151
    and the *Ballet-Fit* workout,
      167–68
    optional, 169–70
Tennessee, schools and universities,
    249
terms, 82–93
    à la seconde, 84
    adagio, 84
    allegro, 84
    attitude, 85
    barre, 85
    cambré, 85
    combination, 86
    croisé, 86
    en bas, 86
    en dedans/en dehors, 88
    en l'air, 88
    en point, 88
    épaulement, 88
    extension, 87

"find your center," 89
fondu, 83
line, 89
marking a combination, 89
pas de chat, 83
port de bras, 83, 90
pull-up, 90
rolling inward (or outward), 91
sickle, 91
sous-sus, 92
supporting leg/working leg, 92
temps de flèche, 83
temps lié, 83
turnout, 92
Texas, schools and universities,
    249–50
third position, 101
tights, 65–67
    "full-fashioned," 66
    recycling, 67
    sculpting, 65–66
    tips on tights, 66–67
tradition, 9–14, 27
turnout, 121
    as a ballet term, 92

U

unitards, 65–67
    "full-fashioned," 66
    recycling, 67
    sculpting, 65–66
Utah, schools and universities, 250

V

video resources, 233–34
Virginia, schools and universities,
    250
Vlhakis, Evie, 53

W

wardrobe, 61–77
    ballet skirts, 70–71
    dance bags, 68–69
    for boys, 71–72
    from your own closet, 63

layering, 64
leg warmers, 67–69
leotards, 63–65
recycling, 67
school regulations, 63
shoes, 72–76
socks, 67
sweatpants and sweatshirts,
    69–70
under wares, 72
unitards, 65–67
See also appearance
warm-up (*Ballet-Fit* workout),
    150–60
    abdominal exercises, 155–56, 156
    demi-pliés, 152
    hamstring stretches, 158
    how much time, 160
    "Kitty Cats," 157
    leg-lifts, 154
    quadriceps stretches, 159
    shoulder raises, 150
    stretches, 152, 153
    taking it slow, 160
    tendus, 151
Washington, schools and universi-
    ties, 250–51
weight
    weight loss and ballet class, 57
    worries concerning, 18
Wisconsin (schools and universi-
    ties), 251

Y

yoga, 2